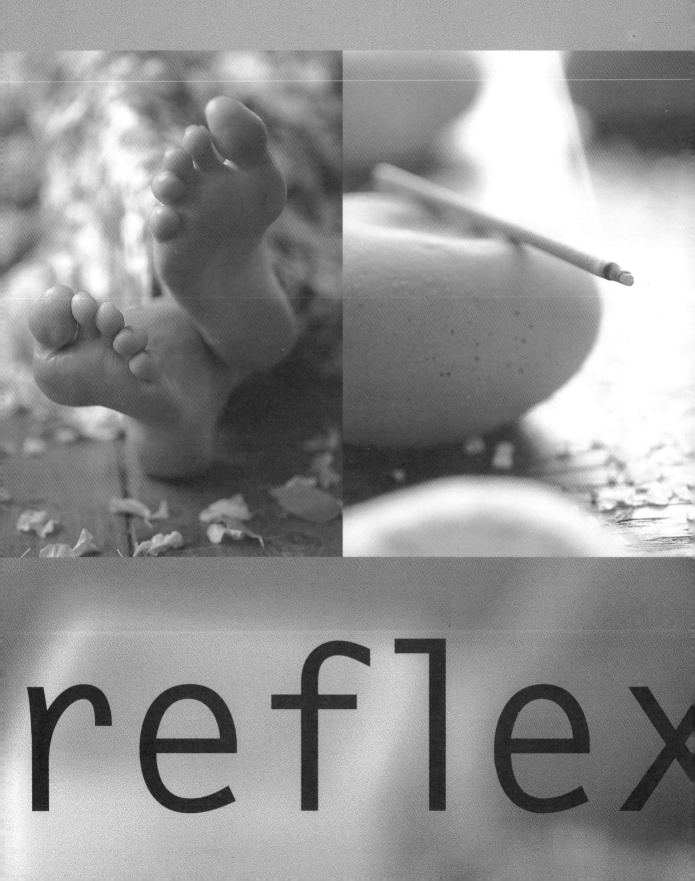

reflex

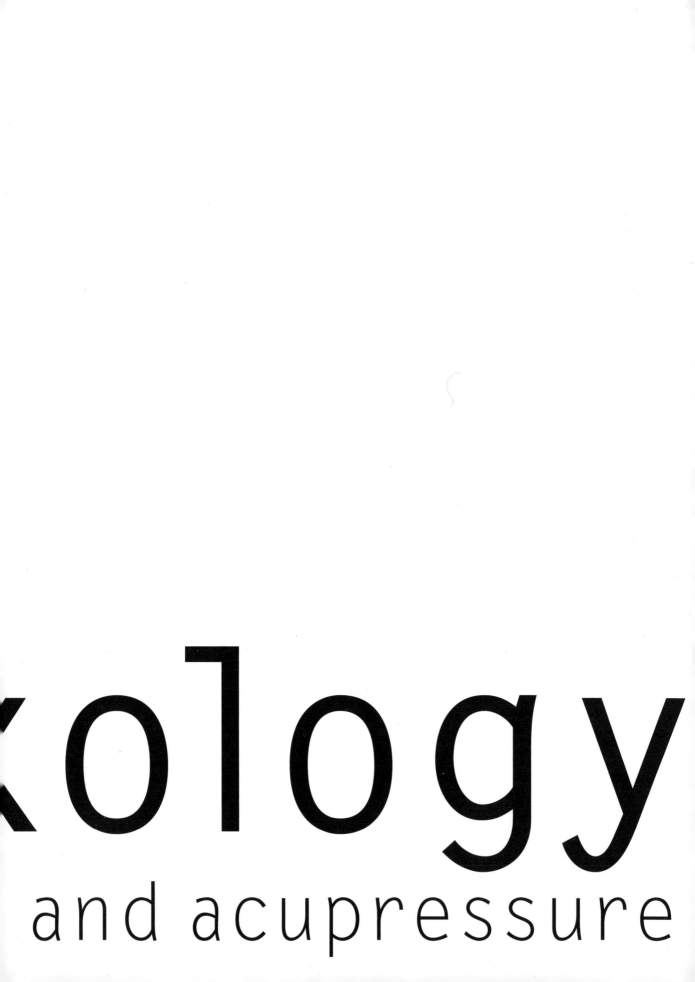

kology
and acupressure

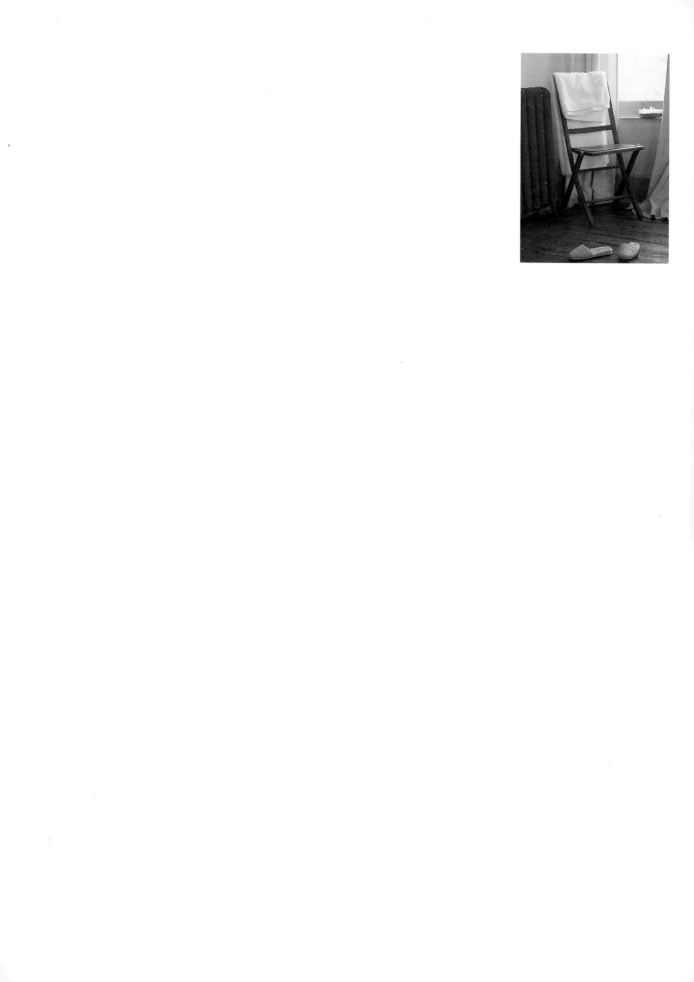

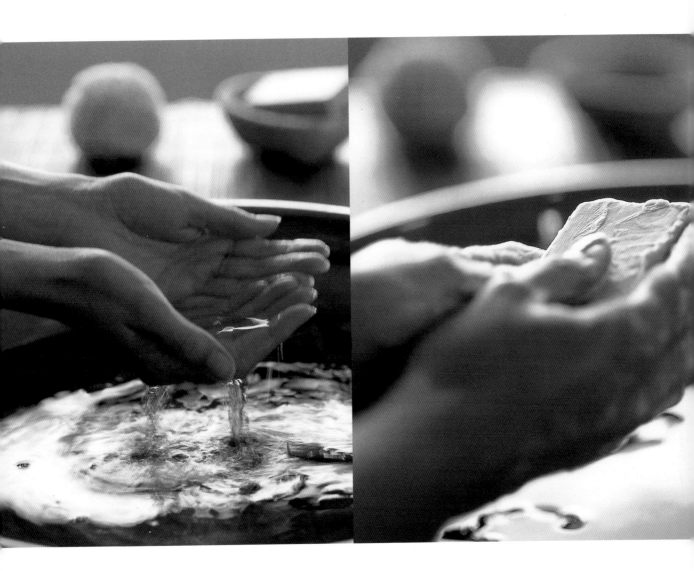

reflexology and acupressure

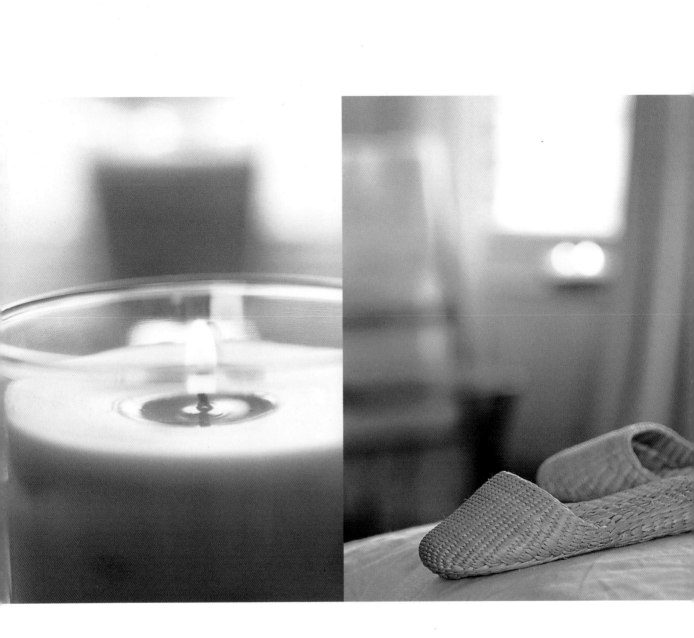

Janet Wright

Consultants:
B.K. Heather and
Sara Mokone

hamlyn

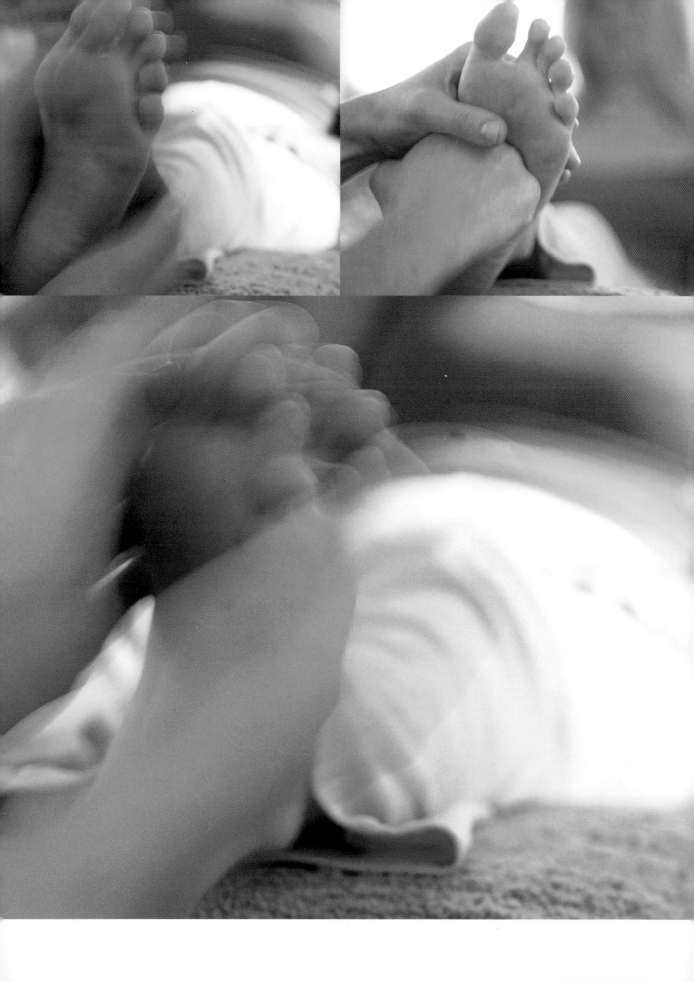

introduction

A hundred years ago no one could have anticipated the dramatic advances that have been made in modern medicine over the past decades. Medical science has found a cure for bubonic plague. It has wiped smallpox, once a mass killer, off the face of the Earth. In the Western world at least, a baby's death is a rare and often unforeseeable tragedy. Yet, at the end of the 20th century and the beginning of the 21st, there has never been more interest in complementary therapies. Why, when orthodox medicine seems to hold the key to all our ills, are we turning away from it in droves?

One answer is that, with each life-saving medical breakthrough, we learn of a new threat to our health. Some of these are caused by the same drugs that save lives. Since the antibiotics that tamed history's most deadly diseases have been used for every trivial infection, new strains of bacteria have evolved which are able to resist them. Side effects from prescription drugs are at least the sixth most common cause of death in the United States. Among hospital patients, about four per cent suffer some new health problem as a result of medical errors, and fourteen per cent of these prove fatal. The figures are thought to be about the same for the United Kingdom.

Other threats to health are caused by wider problems: the stress of our daily lives, air pollution, low-quality mass-produced food, dangerous farming practices and others that damage the environment. We cannot blame medicine for these. At the same time, we cannot expect orthodox medicine to cure them all.

We are even seeing the return of killer diseases we thought had been conquered – tuberculosis, once almost banished by effective drug treatment, is making a frightening comeback, thanks to AIDS and increasing poverty.

Is it any wonder that many people are beginning to feel they are at the mercy of forces beyond their control – and want to regain some measure of power over their lives and their health by seeking a different path? They may do so by looking to practices that in the past have been described as alternative therapies. Among those available, many include at least an element of self-help, which enables people to feel that they can determine their fate to some extent.

Today the terminology for such practices has altered. Whereas the term 'alternative therapies' suggests something to use instead of orthodox medicine, people now think more in terms of 'complementary practices', a term

THE SKELETON

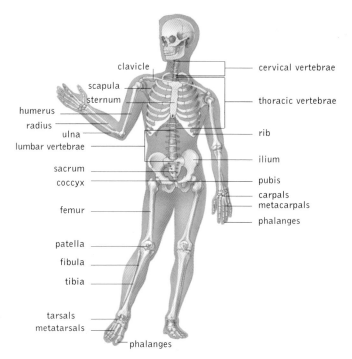

clavicle
cervical vertebrae
scapula
sternum
thoracic vertebrae
humerus
radius
rib
ulna
lumbar vertebrae
ilium
sacrum
coccyx
pubis
carpals
metacarpals
femur
phalanges
patella
fibula
tibia
tarsals
metatarsals
phalanges

THE ENDOCRINE SYSTEM

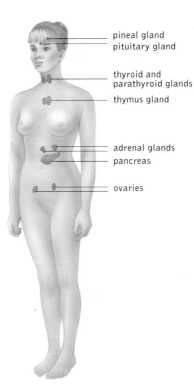

pineal gland
pituitary gland

thyroid and
parathyroid glands

thymus gland

adrenal glands
pancreas

ovaries

THE MAJOR ORGANS

cerebral cortex

upper lungs

heart
lower lungs
spleen
kidneys

liver
stomach
pancreas

small intestine
bladder

large intestine

that incorporates the idea of something extra, which can be used in conjunction with orthodox medicine. A secondary meaning is that these practices 'complement' our own bodily resources, providing the extra help the body may need at a specific time.

We are fortunate today in having a choice about just how natural we want the treatments for our ailments to be. Although we can take antibiotics for serious infections that will not respond to anything else, we may, for example, take a homeopathic remedy to ease a sore throat. Broken bones may need surgery, but if we suffer from back pain we can seek help from a physiotherapist, chiropractor or osteopath.

Increasingly, people are also trying gentle self-help therapies to cure minor ailments or relieve the discomforts of long-term problems. So, when orthodox medicine fails, many people are discovering the power of other therapies, such as reflexology and acupressure, to help in treating their physical and emotional problems.

Above: The illustrations shown here are intended as a guide to be used alongside anatomical references made within the book.

Both reflexology and acupressure are pressure point practices, which are of interest to people who like the idea of learning self-help techniques. They are practical, hands-on therapies with down-to-earth applications in everyday life. Reflexology and acupressure are also linked by their common use of the body's energy centres – a concept that has not yet been recognised by practitioners of Western science, although it is an essential part of a world-wide healing tradition.

Now that the glamour of miracle drugs has been tarnished by their long list of sometimes fatal side effects and adverse reactions, people are looking towards reputable alternative treatments that will not let them down. For many people, Eastern philosophies – and the practices that have evolved from these and from similar traditions – offer this less harmful, more healing approach to ailments and to the maintenance of health.

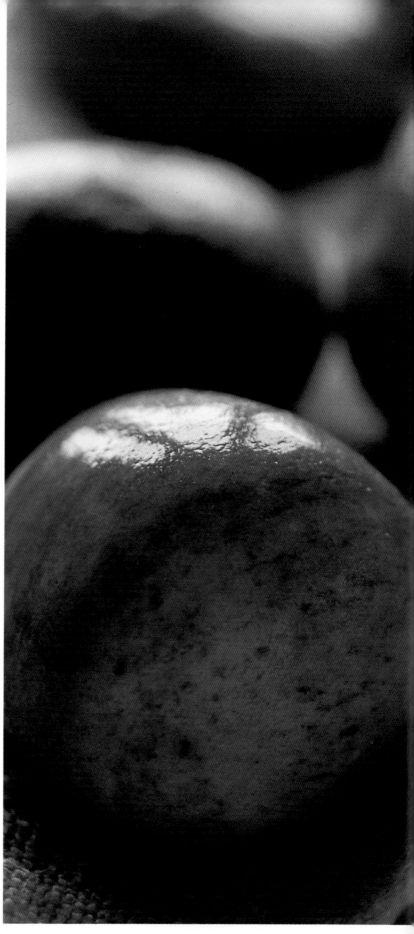

chapter one: basic concepts

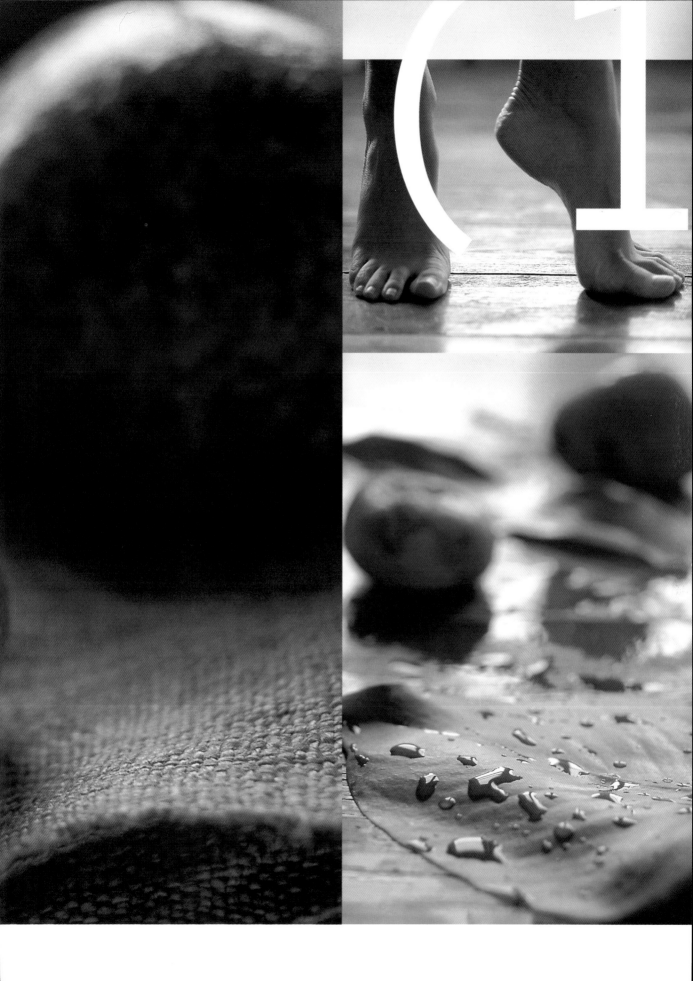

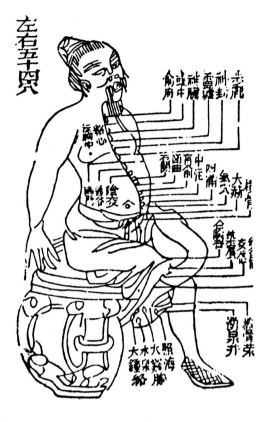

足少陰腎經

左右五十四穴

Above: The Eastern theory of meridian lines that transfer chi around the body is the foundation of acupressure. Here we see the acupoints of the kidney meridian.

TREATING THE WHOLE PERSON

Orthodox medicine identifies an invader (bacteria, a virus or a parasite) or a disorder within the body (such as cancer or hardened arteries) and attacks this 'enemy' with powerful weapons. It deals with individual portions of the body in isolation. Although doctors now recognise some exacerbating factors such as smoking or a high-fat diet, they normally view diseases as events that occur through chance infection – and their offensive tactics often defeat the invader very successfully. Orthodox medicine is based on an in-depth knowledge of physical anatomy and physiology, and on observations of the effects that drugs and surgery have on ailments.

Eastern therapeutic practices – and reflexology, which comes from the same tradition – take what seems to be a less aggressive approach. They believe that an illness is caused by a number of factors, including an inner problem that has weakened the body's natural defences. They seek to heal this by strengthening the body, removing any obstacles to well-being and improving the energy flow. That is not to say that Eastern therapeutic practices are necessarily gentle. Acupuncture can be as invasive as minor surgery; the herbal mixtures used in Chinese herbal medicine can taste foul; some forms of oriental massage make you feel as if holes are being drilled in your bones.

However, everything is aimed at strengthening and healing the whole self (often including non-physical levels such as the spiritual and emotional) rather than simply identifying and attacking certain unwanted symptoms.

Reflexologists and Chinese medical practitioners will work on the symptoms as well, to make the patient more comfortable while dealing with the deeper problem. What they don't do is work on the symptoms alone, since suppressing the symptoms will simply force the problem to express itself in some other way. If you continually suppress the symptoms without tackling the root problem, the ailment will go on getting worse, causing ever more serious effects and finally damaging the entire system. In the same way, no GP would treat the outward symptoms of a serious infection without prescribing drugs to clear the infection itself. However, until very recently, orthodox medicine has not recognised that diseases can stem from more subtle agents than bacteria, viruses and parasites.

ENERGY CHANNELS

The aim of Eastern medicine is to work with the body's strengths and tendencies and with its natural inclination to heal. It is based on a totally different view of what makes humans work – a belief that we run on 'vital energy'. This energy – called prana in India, chi or qi (pronounced 'chee') in China and ki ('kee') in Japan – is carried to every part of the body in a system of channels called meridians, much as the blood is carried to and from the heart in veins and arteries. By massaging an acupressure point on a meridian line – or by inserting an acupuncture needle or burning moxa herbs on the appropriate point – practitioners can affect the movement of chi. Working on the right spot can free trapped chi, slow it down if it is moving too fast or encourage it into an area that it has been bypassing.

There is one major difference between the Western and Eastern systems: you can dissect a human body and reveal the veins and arteries, but you could never see the meridians under a microscope or take a sample of chi for analysis. Like emotions or the soul, our life force exists at a level we cannot see.

This may sound fanciful. However, versions of this system have been operating for thousands of years in many parts of the world, and scientists testing them with modern research methods are finding evidence that they work.

The Chinese system of meridians is not the only body map that differs from our Western model. Reflexologists work on the basis that the body is divided into 10 vertical zones, starting from the top of the head, branching out to end in the 10 fingers, with the main branches ending in the

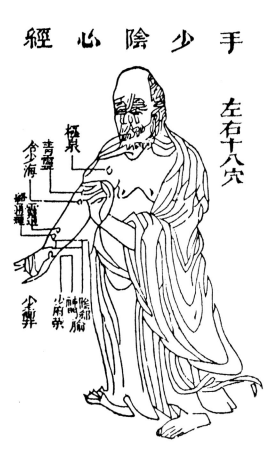

Above: This ancient Chinese body map depicts the acupoints of the heart meridian.
Below: This pulse points diagram is central to the traditional Chinese practitioners' theory of diagnosis.

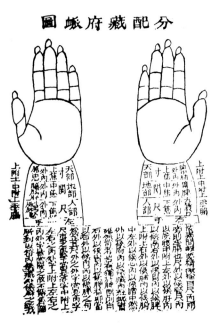

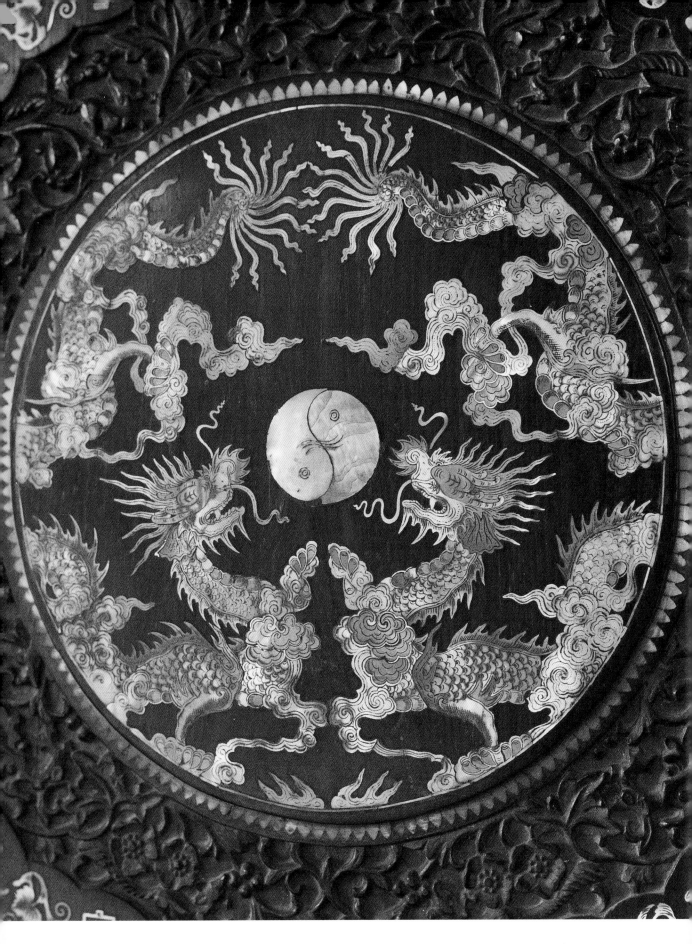

toes. According to this system, each part of the body is represented by a reflex point on the foot or the hand. Another branch of reflexology finds them represented on the ear. This is not contradictory: the original theorists identified reflex points on various parts of the body, but they concentrated on those which they found were the most powerful.

Like acupressurists, reflexologists aim to help the body's energy circulate effectively without blockages, energy loss or stagnation. In putting imbalances right, they hope to stimulate the body's healing processes and, preferably, to prevent illness from developing. Reflexology has been found useful for stress-related conditions such as allergies, asthma, insomnia, depression, anxiety and migraine; disorders caused by muscle tension such as back pain and fibrositis; and women's conditions such as PMS, pregnancy, childbirth and menopause. It has eased the symptoms of chronic fatigue syndrome (CFS), multiple sclerosis and even cancer.

Some reflexologists even use the meridian system as well as the zones. They believe reflexology works by stimulating the six meridians that begin or end in the feet. And although modern reflexology was developed by people who did not know the Chinese system, there are startling similarities. For example, there is a powerful point on the bottom of the ball of the foot, right in the centre, which reflexologists call the solar plexus point. This is a major reflex point for working on stress and replenishing energy. Acupressurists know it as the 'bubbling spring', the first point on the kidney meridian, which carries the energy we are born with; this spot is used for calming distress and dizziness. In the Indian tradition, incidentally, this is the Earth chakra, which balances the whole body.

KEEPING YOUR BALANCE

To a Chinese practitioner, the balance of various elements is also important, especially yin and yang – opposite forces that complement each other. Yin and yang are sometimes described as the female and male energies, but that is an oversimplification. Each of us contains both. Yin energy is connected with what is receptive, restful, cool, ingoing, dark and soft. Yang energy is forceful, active, warm, outgoing, light, hard and so on. Too much yin or yang energy is unhealthy for either sex: we need a balance of the two to create healthy chi and prevent illness.

In this book we will not go into that kind of detail. However, it is relevant here because it shows how much emphasis practitioners of energy medicine place on keeping things in balance – something about which modern health educators are now trying to persuade us.

Left: This 19th-century Vietnamese inlay depicts the yin-yang pearl guarded by Imperial dragons.
Below: This Song Dynasty painting shows a moxibustion treatment – a method of stimulating pressure points with herbs.

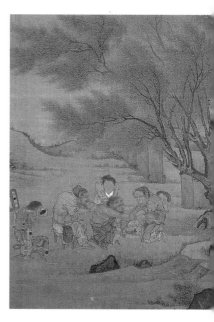

According to this outlook, disease is caused by some kind of imbalance, or by a problem with energy in a particular area: eiher too much or too little or a blockage in its circulation.

MIND AND BODY

Western doctors are just starting to get to grips with a phenomenon called psychoneuroimmunology (PNI) – the effect mind and body can have on each other. This is a huge new area of study, looking at things that may seem baffling to a 21st-century Western individual. We have been brought up to believe our bodies run like machines, sometimes going wrong and needing repairs, but not affected by outside forces other than accidents or the wrong fuel. Yet broad-minded doctors have accepted that some cases don't seem to fit into this framework.

The new field of PNI is turning up evidence that our emotions play a vital role in our physical health. This is no surprise to reflexologists. Like many complementary practitioners, they have always been clear about the role emotions play in healing or harming us. Depression and anger are the best known problems. However, all kinds of emotion can tip the balance.

Some of the effects of PNI are so obvious and immediate that they are unquestionable. How many times have you been so worried about an intractable problem that you have ended up with a splitting headache? And if you are feeling angry or upset when you're eating, the resulting bout of indigestion is not totally unexpected.

No wonder people use expressions such as 'My boss is a pain in the neck', or even 'she makes me sick' – they are quite literally true. It is the same when you are feeling 'down-hearted'; grief can feel like a weight around your heart. A sense of tightness in the chest is a common symptom of anxiety, sometimes leading to frightening pains that make people fear a heart attack.

Now researchers are starting to admit that we respond to forces that just don't fit the mechanical model. Studies have revealed that our gut feelings were right. On the one hand, bereavement can lead to cancer and a woman's risk of breast cancer doubles during the year after her marriage breaks up. Frustration can affect the working of our intestines. Anger and depression increase the risk of heart disease.

On the other hand, researchers have also found that laughter strengthens the immune system and that people who go to religious services tend to live longer. When people do develop a life-threatening disease, a loving marriage is one of their best aids to recovery. Sick people with a close circle of friends and family are more likely to recover, and not just because they are being looked after. They do better than those whose material needs are met by professional carers.

Reflexologists believe that working on the zones, through the feet or hands, helps to harmonise all our systems – mental and emotional as well as physical. And because reflexology as we know it was developed during the 20th century, it recognises the role played by that modern bugbear, stress.

STRESS AND HEALTH

For most of us, life is harder and more uncertain now than it was 20 or 30 years ago. If you grew up expecting that, in general, life got better decade by decade, it is a shock to find jobs disappearing, benefits cut, prospects evaporating and health services shrinking away. Insecurity and powerlessness are major causes of stress, so it is not surprising that so many of us suffer from it.

While it is important to tackle the causes of stress, hands-on energy-moving practices such as reflexology or acupressure can do much to help. They can ease the symptoms, giving you more strength to work on your problems. The very act of stopping what you are doing in order to work on your pressure points – or having someone give you a treatment – can be calming. These practices are also believed to free the flow of energy through the body where these have been restricted by emotional upheaval.

A good reflexology treatment can be deeply relaxing, allowing tension to ebb out of the entire body. Muscles loosen up and the blood circulates more freely, bringing nutrients to every cell in the body. Reflexologists work on specific pressure points to counteract stress and to bolster the body's immune system against its ill-effects. In addition, any kind of massage can relieve stress. The long strokes used in reflexology are as important, from this point of view, as is the work on pressure points.

THE VIEW FROM CHINA

Acupressurists work on an even more direct link between emotion and physical illness than reflexologists. Chinese traditional medical theory holds that each emotion is linked with one of the organs; the emotion can affect the working of that organ and its related meridian.

Fear, for example, affects the kidneys and the kidney meridian. 'Fear' covers a multitude of unpleasant feelings, from timidity to the pervasive modern problem of free-floating anxiety, common among people who have lost confidence in their ability to deal with the world. The results may be what we'd expect of fear – symptoms such as heart palpitations, dry mouth and, in children,

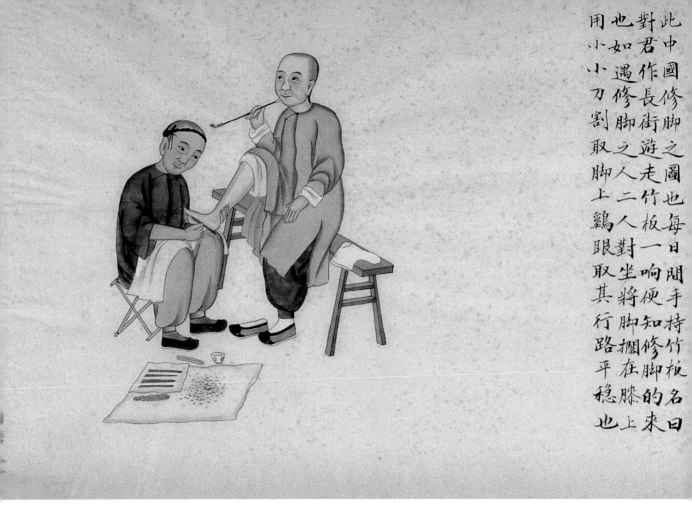

此中國修脚之圖也每日閒手持竹板名曰
對君作長街遊走竹板一响便知修脚的來
也如遇修脚之人二人對坐將脚擱在膝上
用小小刀割取脚上鷄眼取其行路平穩也

Above: A 19th-century print depicting a foot massage. This type of massage has been common in China for centuries.

bed-wetting. However, since the Chinese see these as resulting from depleted kidney energy, they treat the problem by working on that meridian rather than prescribing heart drugs or just cutting down on drinks before bedtime. Enlightened practitioners in the East or West will also recommend dealing with the causes of fear.

Grief is linked with the lungs and through them can affect the heart. Worry can also reduce lung energy and lead on to breathlessness and feelings of anxiety. Overwork puts a strain on the spleen, reducing its ability to keep the digestive system working at peak efficiency. Shock causes a sudden drop in heart chi – with direct effects on the heart such as palpitations – but can also reduce kidney energy. Anger can create an excess of liver energy, causing headaches and dizziness. Long-term anger (which can take the form of nagging resentment, frustration and even depression as well as the more obvious irritability) can make this excessive liver energy interfere with the spleen's work of protecting the digestive system.

Enjoyable emotions such as happiness are good for the body as well as the mind. Yet too much can overstimulate the heart, causing restlessness and insomnia. Once again, it is the oriental rule of 'moderation in all things'.

Energy medicine is part of a rich healing

tradition that has developed, in various forms

and at various times, around the world. We

have no way of telling whether travellers took

the knowledge and practice of energy

medicine from one part of the world to

another long before records were made of

such movements. However, there is no logical

reason, either, why different cultures should

not have developed similar ideas and

practices independently.

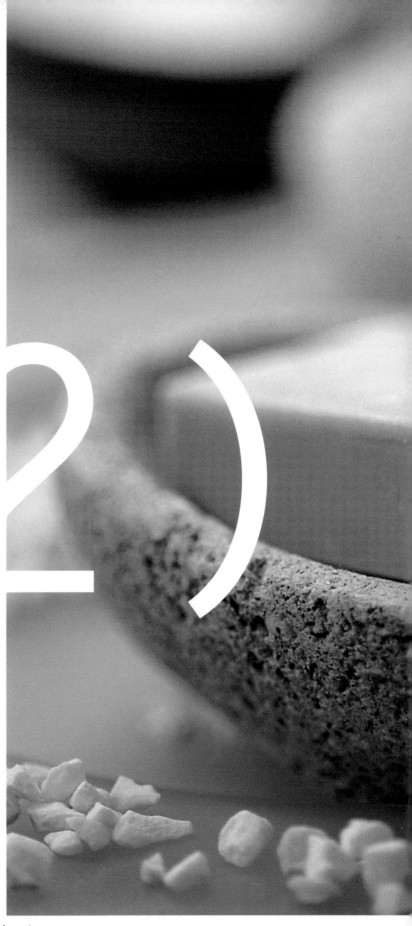

chapter two: history

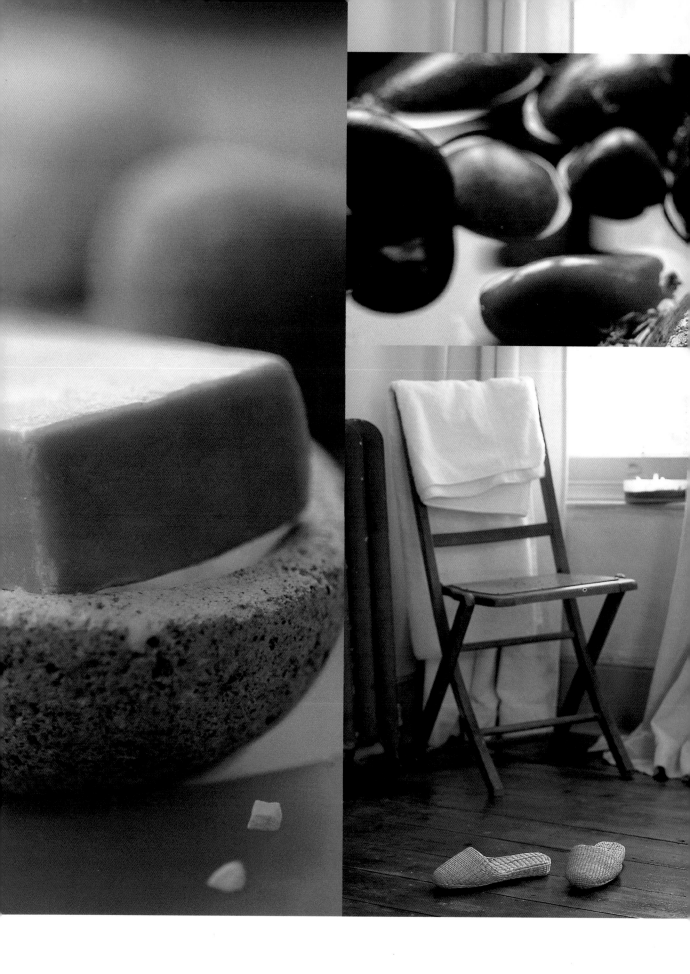

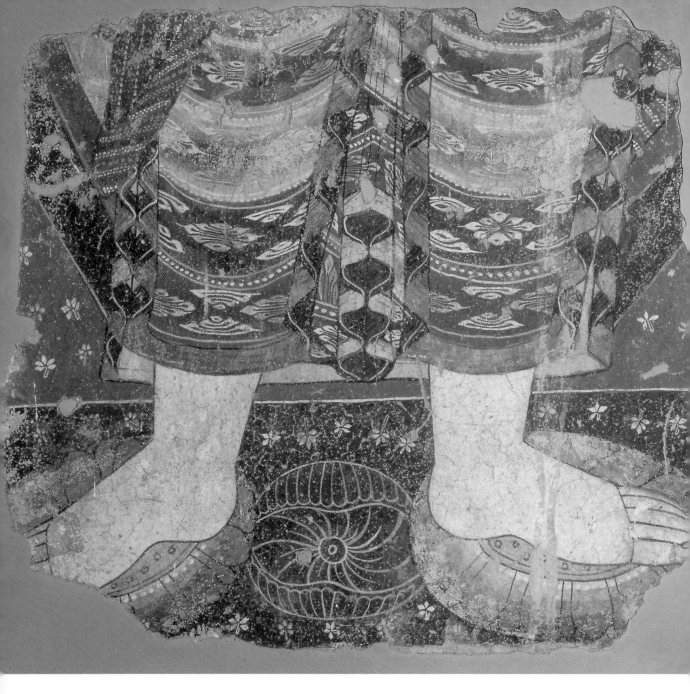

Above: Fragment of an Indian wall painting of the Buddha, showing his robe and feet. The painting has been dated to the 7–8th centuries. It is possible that reflexology originates from India.

BEGINNINGS

Motivated, possibly, by the instinct to ease pain, or through a chance discovery, our distant ancestors would have noted what appeared to be an effective treatment and tried to produce the same effect again when a similar problem arose. Without our armoury of drugs and surgical techniques, and before healing became specialised enough to employ people full time, they had to find methods they could use on themselves. Lacking detailed knowledge of the body's physiological processes, they had to rely on subtle observations.

Indian traditional medicine, Ayurveda, includes work on the body's energies. Ancient Greek medical theories (from which orthodox Western medicine developed) also included a system of body energies, although this later fell out of favour. Acupressure is part of the Chinese tradition, which is particularly well documented and highly evolved, having developed continuously over a period of more than 3000 years.

Feet and hands, two hard-working parts of the body, have always been popular sites for massage. There is an element of loving care in this treatment, which undoubtedly plays a role of its own in the process of healing and relieving pain. In the Christian tradition, Jesus insists on washing his apostles' feet. Pictures and references to foot massage abound throughout the world, although we have no way of knowing exactly what techniques were used.

The earliest definite medical reference comes from Ancient Egypt around 2500 BC. A wall carving in the tomb of the renowned doctor Ankhmahor shows doctors working on their patients' hands and feet. The fact that hieroglyphics show the patient is saying 'Don't do anything that hurts' confirms that this is a medical technique, and not a beauty treatment or relaxing massage.

Japanese practitioners of a branch of reflexology called sokushinjutsu believe their therapy was first used in India some 5000 years ago, taken to China by Buddhist monks some time after the 3rd century BC, and on to Japan. Reflexology historian Christine Issel has noticed that traditional paintings of the feet of the Hindu god Vishnu are covered in symbols coinciding with reflex points.

Before the arrival of the Buddhist monks, the Chinese were using their own form of foot therapy. In the 4th century BC, a Chinese doctor called Wang Wei used to insert acupuncture needles at relevant points on his patients' bodies, then apply firm thumb pressure to the soles of their feet in order to release healing energy. Foot massage, and methods of diagnosis by means of observation of the feet, were recorded in China over the next few hundred years.

Healers in North and South America are believed to have worked on people's feet, and a form of zone therapy – using pressure on one part of the body to relieve pain in another – was recorded in 16th-century Europe. We do not know exactly how these techniques worked; however, by the 19th century British doctors who specialised in disorders of the nervous system had discovered that touching pressure points on various parts of the body could cause numbness and affect the working of internal organs. At the same time, doctors in Germany, where massage was more popular, were discovering that hand massage brought especially potent pain relief.

Reflexology as we know it today was developed in the early 20th century, when an American doctor, William

Below: Knowledge of Eastern therapies may have been brought to the West by adventurers such as Marco Polo, shown here departing from Venice.

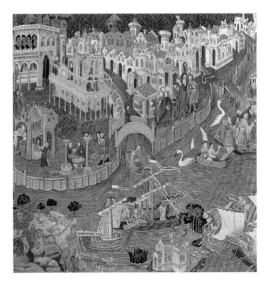

Fitzgerald, worked out a system of pressure points to use for anaesthesia. Having found that these existed all over the body, he developed a system of zones much like those used today, and called this zone therapy. One of his colleagues used to give startling demonstrations by proving he could stick a pin in someone's face without causing pain, after pressing the right spot on the volunteer's hand.

In 1915 Dr Fitzgerald published an article entitled 'To Stop That Toothache, Squeeze Your Toe!' in 'Everybody's Magazine', and in 1917 he published his first book on the subject. However, although the practice was taken up by some doctors and dentists, Fitzgerald's treatment methods remained controversial.

In the 1930s, the American physiotherapist Eunice Ingham discovered that the most powerful reflex points were located in the feet, and she eventually drew up the foot maps that are still in use today. She then concentrated on this area, calling her work 'reflexology' and travelling around the United States to teach it to anyone who wanted to learn. In the 1950s reflexology came under fire as an allegedly fraudulent practice, and several American practitioners were charged with practising medicine without a licence – although they were eventually acquitted.

In 1966 Doreen Bayley introduced reflexology to Britain. An explosion of interest in alternative therapies brought it to a wider audience during the 1970s, when Ann Gillanders set up the British School of Reflexology. Reflexology has become so popular that some GPs now employ reflexologists to give treatments through the National Health Service. In Denmark, reflexology is the most popular of all complementary therapies: about nine per cent of the population have tried it.

THE CHINESE BACKGROUND

Some of the most convincing evidence for energy treatments is the role they play in traditional Chinese medicine, a method of treatment that is massively documented and backed by solid evidence (see 'What the scientists say' on page 29).

Although acupressure is often described as an offshoot of acupuncture, acupressure probably came first. People must have noticed that pressure on certain spots on the body relieved pain. Over time they discovered that applying pressure or heat to the right place could affect the working of internal organs. While a swig of rum or brandy was all the anaesthetic a patient would receive in the West until the 19th century, pain-relief and anaesthesia were among the first uses for acupressure.

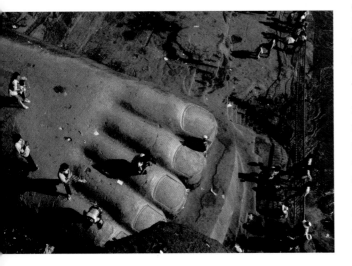

Below: Foot of a colossal seated Buddha on the banks of China's Jiang (Yangzi) River. Reflexology and acupressure have their roots in ancient Chinese medicine.

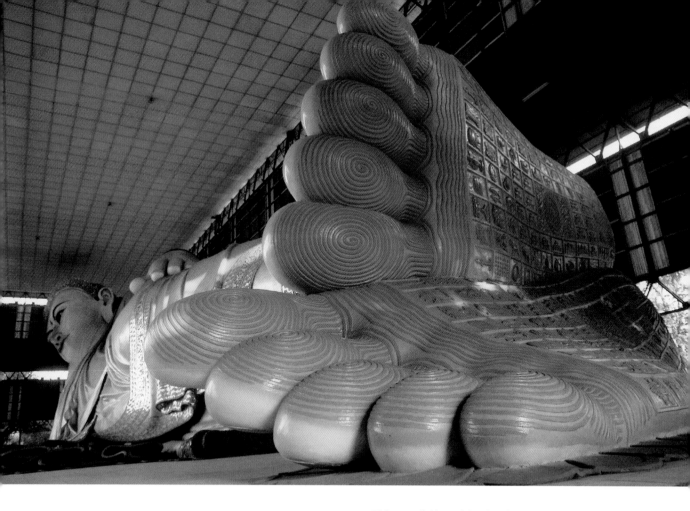

Above: Inscriptions are evident on the soles of the feet of this reclining Buddha. The statue was erected at Pegu, Myanmar (formerly Burma).

This was followed by the discovery that using sharp objects could have an even stronger effect. Before they knew how to work metal, the first acupuncturists were treating pressure points with differently shaped stones, sharpened bones, bamboo slivers and fragments of pottery. Some 2000 years ago Prince Liu Sheng and his wife were buried surrounded by their treasures, including a set of gold and silver acupuncture needles. By the time the 'Canon of Medicine' was written, during the last millennium BC, nine types of needle were in use, ranging from those which were as fine as a hair to a blunt device for applying pressure, and another with an egg-shaped end for massaging the points. Books of the time also refer to the meridian system and to moxibustion, a method of heating pressure points with burning herbs.

Acupuncture/acupressure is just one branch of traditional Chinese medicine. The other branches are herbalism, massage, nutrition and energy-moving exercises such as qigong (chi kung). All of them can work together and complement each other. However, each one is effective on its own; and all of them aim to work on energies as well as on physical factors.

The earliest surviving references to Chinese medicine are about 3000 years old, giving herbal recipes and

recording the effects of weather on people's health. By the
4th century BC, the standard methods of diagnosis had
been recorded – which included listening to the patient.
However, the best preserved and most famous work is the
'Nei Jing', the 'Yellow Emperor's Canon of Medicine' –
also known as the 'Yellow Emperor's Classic of Internal
Medicine'. Supposedly written by China's mythical first
emperor, this was in fact compiled by a number of
scholars some time before the 3rd century BC, with
various notes added over the next few hundred years.
By AD 220, this exhaustive tome encapsulated
everything that was then known about the fields of health
and medicine.

Along with other Chinese works of the same period, the
'Nei Jing' emphasised the importance of cleanliness, good
food and a well-balanced way of life. Moderation was
recommended in all things: food, work, study and sleep.
Fresh air was considered vital for adults and children, as
was a clean water supply – ideas that did not catch on in
the Western world until the 19th century. (In the 12th
century, some 700 years before doctors in the West could
be persuaded to wash their hands between dissecting
corpses and delivering babies, 'The New Book on Child
Care' insisted that scissors should be sterilised with fire
before cutting the umbilical cord.)

Central to the medical philosophy that was revealed by
these ancient texts was the importance of keeping the
body's energies in balance.

'All types of disease may occur when one is over-
exposed to wind, rain, cold or heat; also when there is
imbalance of yin and yang; or in extreme joy or anger,
with irregular eating, undesirable living conditions, or
in a state of fright or dread,' the 'Canon of Medicine'
pointed out. At the time, it was a battle to convince
people that disease was caused by these preventable
factors, rather than by vengeful gods. The book
comments, rather testily, 'It is no use to talk about
medical principles with persons who believe in ghosts
and spirits; neither is there any way to discuss medical
techniques with persons who oppose acupuncture, surgery
and medicinal substances.'

In the 2nd and 3rd centuries AD exercises were invented
that later developed into tai chi (tai ji quan). Based on the
movements of five animals – tiger, deer, bear, monkey and
bird – the exercises were designed to build a robust
constitution by moving energies and keeping the body
strong and supple.

The system grew increasingly sophisticated as the
centuries passed, yet the main elements were already in
practice from the beginning. Although diseases were

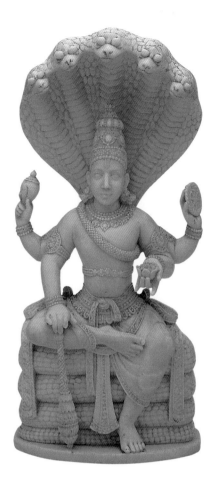

Above: **The Hindu god Vishnu is often
portrayed wtih symbols on his feet that
correspond to reflex points.**

treated with an impressive armoury of herbs and surgical techniques, medicine's main role was preventive.

As the author of the 'Canon of Medicine' warned his readers: 'A wise doctor does not cure a disease, but prevents the disease. A wise statesman never brings peace to his country, but always keeps his country in peace. If the doctor waits until the disease develops to treat it, or a statesman who administers his country waits until it is in turbulence, it will be too late. It is equivalent to opening a well when one is already thirsty, or forging weapons after the war has started.'

The Chinese enthusiasm for knowledge was not matched by any enthusiasm for travel, so no one took China's discoveries to the rest of the world. However, because China has been a cultural centre for thousands of years, visitors from neighbouring countries have taken the philosophy home with them, where it has evolved in local forms. Japanese scholars, immersed in Chinese culture, learned the Chinese medical system and developed their own version of acupressure which is known as shiatsu.

The traveller Marco Polo wrote admiringly about the Chinese health system during the 12th century, but without usable details. Garbled news of acupuncture reached the West through an employee of the Dutch East India company in the 17th century. Unfortunately he mistook the meridians shown on the traditional Chinese medical charts for veins and arteries, which must have baffled his audience. A Dutch doctor wrote a treatise on acupuncture in 1883, but information about Chinese medicine did not become widely available in Europe until as late as the 20th century.

Most of the Chinese medical theory makes absolute sense to the modern Western eye. The insistence on moderation, wholesome food and hygiene (for doctors as well as patients) remained far in advance of Western medical practice until little more than a century ago.

Herbal medicines do not seem too strange to someone used to modern drugs, especially since herbalism was widely practised in Europe until a few hundred years ago and is now enjoying a popular revival. The benefits of Chinese herbal medicine have recently begun to be reported in international publications after double-blind, placebo-controlled trials, and its efficacy was noted in a report in the 'British Medical Journal' in 1997. (See 'What the scientists say' page 29.)

As far as the meridian system is concerned, there is enough published evidence that something is working in this regard to counteract the natural scepticism of Western thinking.

Below: Attendants massage the feet and hands of the pharaoh Ptahhotep II in this relief dated to c. 2350 BC. Some of the earliest records of medical treatment come from Ancient Egypt.

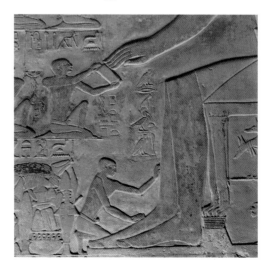

As drug-free, hands-on therapies, reflexology and acupressure are ideal for self-help. They lend themselves to easing both long-term conditions and sudden crises, and are suitable as a supporting, complementary back-up to orthodox medical treatment or as first aid where this is relevant. Reflexology and acupressure can also be used to treat friends and family. Two groups of people who can gain particular benefit from these techniques are children and the elderly.

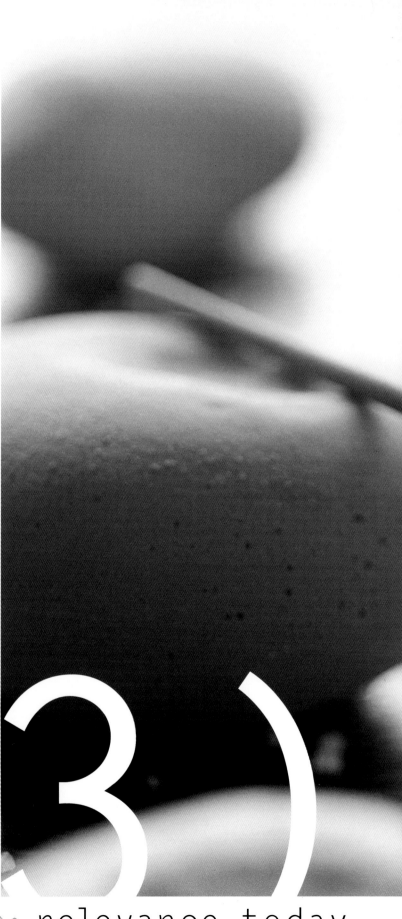

chapter three: relevance today

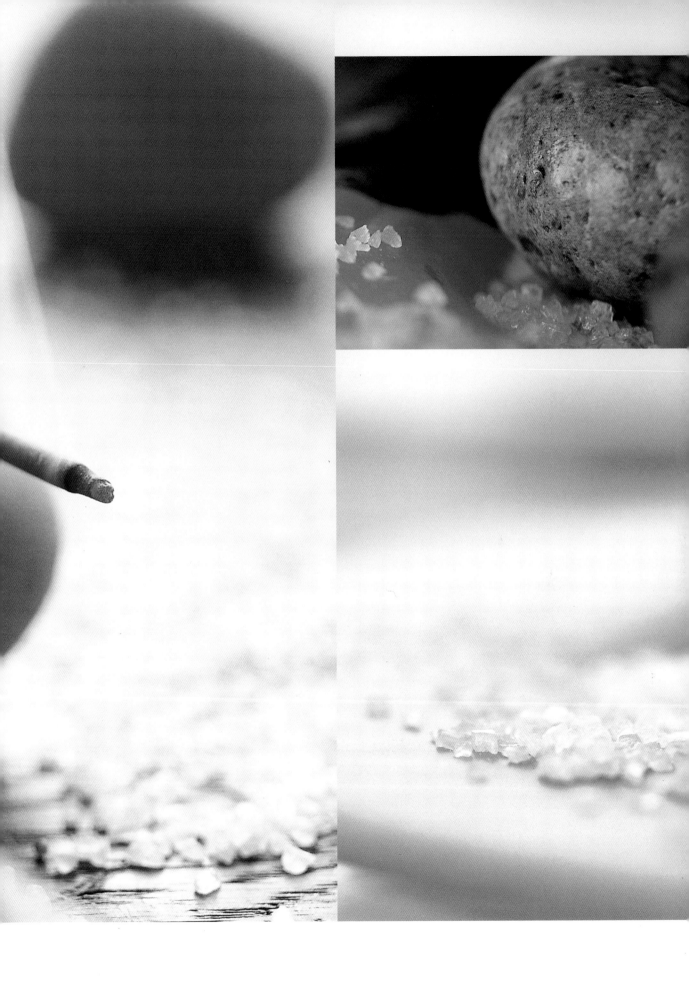

CHILDREN

Children often respond quickly to these gentle treatments. No parent wants to keep taking a child back to the GP with minor ailments, running the risk of picking up new infections in the waiting room and going home with a shopping list of drugs. (In any case, doctors have found that some children's ailments, for example ear infections, tend to clear up as quickly without antibiotics as with them, and antibiotics have no effect at all on most sore throats, since these are rarely caused by bacteria.) Yet to be fair to overworked GPs, they don't like handing out drugs, especially to children. However, they have little time to spend with each patient – and, frequently, parents feel that their child has not had proper treatment if they leave without a prescription.

Small children respond particularly well to reflexology and acupressure because they have not yet learned our deep cultural dislike of being touched. Anyone travelling around the world will notice that in many countries adults of both sexes are more tactile, touching each other while they are talking, draping an arm around a friend or squashing cheerfully together on bus seats. We are the odd ones out at this. Because we have so little non-sexual physical contact, we tend to associate touch with either violence or sex: one frightening and the other inappropriate in the wrong circumstances.

However, children are still citizens of the world. They have not yet learned to feel uncomfortable with a human touch. Still at home with their bodies, they are not likely to object to a soothing touch that doesn't hurt and could possibly help. Child and baby massage is practised in many parts of the world to promote general good health and well-being. With a child small enough to fall asleep in your arms, the combination of a pressure point treatment and some long calming massage strokes may be all that is needed. Older children can learn some of the techniques themselves. They don't need to understand the theory; they are fascinated by discovering how different parts of the body link up.

Remember, though: don't hesitate to take your child to a doctor if your child is ill and the problem gets worse, especially if the child has a high temperature or is suffering from a headache and stiff neck (which in rare but important cases can be a sign of meningitis).

THE ELDERLY

For the elderly, reflexology and acupressure provide two important benefits in addition to the healing effects. As a society we have little respect for old age. Retired people

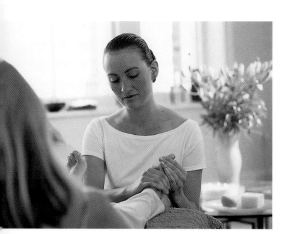

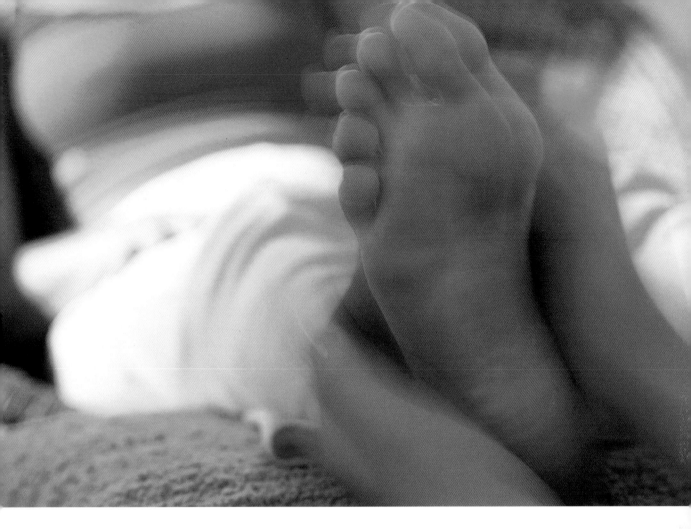

hear politicians moaning about the cost of pensions and see the public services they now need to use being steadily cut back. The thrifty, honest virtues their generation grew up with are now belittled and their cooperative values, forged during difficult times, are considered out of date. In many cultures their experience is highly valued, but in the West people seem to lose their worth once they have stopped working.

Having someone take the time to give them a treatment can remind an elderly person that they are valued. Acupressure and reflexology are also ideal techniques for a less active person to learn. Anyone whose hands are not arthritic or damaged by diabetes can try them. Both receiving treatment and having a skill to offer others provide a natural psychological boost.

While many elderly people would not feel comfortable with a full massage, they could enjoy the healing benefits of some reflexology or acupressure techniques. Treatments on the hands, face and shoulders may be the most enjoyable. However, when giving treatment, do bear in mind that the skin of older people becomes fragile and that their bones become brittle, so don't do anything that could cause pain or injury.

People suffering from diabetes – which many develop as they get older – need special care for their feet, since their circulation becomes less efficient. So if you are caring for a relative with diabetes, some very gentle reflexology could form part of their foot care routine. Concentrate on the soothing strokes and remember that the skin may be slightly numb, so you can't rely on a yelp of pain to warn you that you are pressing too hard.

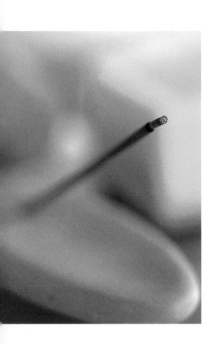

LEARNING THE TECHNIQUES

Anyone can learn and use self-help techniques such as acupressure and reflexology. It is up to you how far you want to take it. This book offers a full reflexology treatment and enough acupressure training to deal with everyday problems. You could take it further and go on a short course to improve your skills and ensure all your movements are correct – no book can teach that as well as a qualified instructor running a course.

Having some professional treatments is also well worth the money. Although you can choose either reflexology or acupressure to relieve symptoms, both are holistic therapies; what they are really good at is balancing your whole system. You may find the problems you have been treating yourself have other aspects you had not thought of, which a professional can quickly pick up. Many practitioners are happy to give you guidance on self-help maintenance routines to practise between sessions.

To find a qualified practitioner, ask friends if they can recommend anyone, or send a stamped addressed envelope to a reputable organisation (see Useful Addresses on page 124). When you contact a practitioner, before making an appointment ask how much they charge and whether they will expect you to have a series of treatments. Some acupuncturists also practise acupressure, but if you are thinking of having acupuncture treatment it is particularly important to make sure that the practitioner is qualified and uses sterile needles.

WORKING MIRACLES?

In using complementary therapies, we are taking responsibility for our own well-being. That is not to say we are going to refuse a life-saving drug or healing surgery – or even an aspirin to dismiss an intractable headache. It means we are weaning ourselves off the idea that illness is something that just happens by chance and is cured by a prescription from the G.P.

Taking responsibility for your health includes listening to what doctors say – they spent a lot of time training for their work. Whatever you feel about some of the drugs they prescribe, they are the experts when it comes to diagnosis. Remember too that therapies such as reflexology and acupressure work alongside orthodox medical treatments and may enhance their effects. It's not an either/or situation.

Taking this responsibility also includes taking whatever steps you need to improve your health in other ways. It goes without saying that smoking is bad for your general health, and not just your heart and lungs. Drinking too much alcohol is also harmful, especially if you have slipped into having a drink every day. You can also become addicted to caffeine, from cola drinks as well as tea and coffee. Your daily diet should include as few processed foods as possible; the majority should be a selection of fresh vegetables, fruit and cereals (including bread) with some protein foods such as fish, meat, dairy or vegetarian products such as tofu or Quorn. Processed foods are generally high in the most harmful form of fat and low in necessary nutritional ingredients. They are fine as the odd snack or treat, but they should not form the basis of your diet.

Today only a small proportion of the population gets a healthy amount of exercise through their daily activities. At least three times a week you need to take half an hour's exercise, enough to raise your heart rate so you are just slightly puffed but can still talk without gasping.

Our attitudes and outlook also play a vital role in maintaining health. Negative thoughts do more than bring us down. If you slip into the habits of resentment, regret for the past, envy, jealousy or despair (for they are habits) they will drag you into depression and lethargy. These can eventually damage the immune system and may lead to physical illness.

Taking responsibility for ourselves is empowering, although it is important not to become unrealistic and expect to work miracles. Complementary practitioners do not possess supernatural powers, and neither do we. What we do have is a chance to make healthy choices, take an empowering attitude and give ourselves the best life we can. On an everyday level we can make significant changes in our health and well-being. It is worth the effort, because we are worth it.

WHAT THE SCIENTISTS SAY

Every practitioner has stories to tell about the amazing effects of reflexology or acupressure. These personal accounts are valuable indications of their benefits. However, scientists, quite reasonably, like to prove things with standardised experiments that can be matched against other similar tests.

The most convincing of these is the placebo-controlled trial, one in which volunteers agree to take, for example, a tablet every day, without knowing whether it is a drug or a 'placebo', a harmless sugar pill with no medicinal effects. Researchers check the results from both groups, those who have taken the drug and those on the placebo. In this way they can evaluate the genuine effects of the drug on the first group of volunteers and any improvements in those taking the placebo. Improvements in the placebo group may be a result of the body's natural healing processes, for example, or because taking part in the trial has given

them a helpful psychological boost.

Most highly rated of all is the double-blind placebo-controlled trial, in which even the people giving out the pills don't know who is taking a placebo and who is taking the drug – so they cannot accidentally influence the patient in any way.

When scientists complain there is little solid evidence in favour of complementary practices, they mean that few have proved themselves in double-blind placebo-controlled trials. However, these experiments were formulated to test the efficacy of drugs. In many cases such tests are simply not suitable for complementary practices. The argument put forth by many complementary practitioners is that their techniques are tailored for the individual and do not consist of standard routines. They also question whether it matters if some of the benefits their patients feel come from the caring treatment and the patient's trust in the practitioner, both of which are part of the healing effect. Therefore they do not care to take part in trials which they consider inappropriate.

It is now accepted that the mind has powerful effects on the body, so some of the physical benefits of both orthodox and complementary medicine are likely to stem from the psychological value of being looked after. In the case of complementary medicine, the practitioner's own energies may also affect the results of any energy-moving therapy. Because of this it is difficult to test a 'fake' treatment against the genuine one, since even the fake treatment is almost certain to do some good.

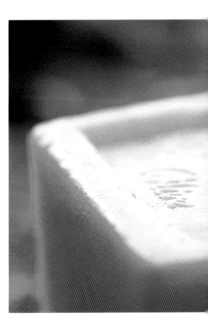

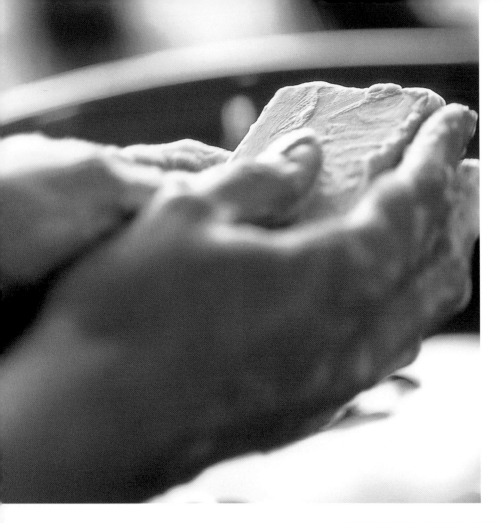

PUTTING IT TO THE TEST

Despite the obstacles to scientific research, energy-moving therapies have been tested and found successful. Reflexology – like all forms of massage – is known to improve the circulation of blood and of lymph, the fluid that carries toxins out of the body. However, recent experiments seem to show effects that could not be ascribed to improved circulation alone.

For example, Chinese researchers tested two groups of volunteers with diabetes. All of them continued taking their usual drugs, but one group was also treated with reflexology. The result was that in the latter group blood-sugar levels became much steadier than they did among those in the first group.

In another study, American reflexologist Bill Flocco persuaded 52 women suffering from PMS to keep diaries of their symptoms over six months. Part of this group received reflexology during this period, and the remainder received what they were told was reflexology but was in fact merely pressure on irrelevant parts of their feet. The first group reported nearly twice as much relief from the psychological upheaval of PMS as the second, and nearly three times more improvement in physical symptoms.

Senior lecturer Deborah Botting, of the University of Glamorgan's Nurse Education Centre, read through dozens of reflexology research papers and found some that, despite all the difficulties, seemed to meet the criteria for a well-conducted trial. In one of these, volunteers with lower back pain received either real or fake reflexology while continuing with their usual medication and physiotherapy. Those who had the genuine treatment had so much less pain and more mobility that many were able to give up their pain-killing drugs. However, as she points out in her article 'Review of Literature on the Effectiveness of Reflexology' in the journal 'Complementary Therapies in Nursing and Midwifery', (Number 3, 1997), more research needs to be done – and made widely available.

There is no shortage of research into traditional Chinese medicine, and Western researchers have been surprised to find it stands up to scientific scrutiny. Herbal remedies are the easiest to test in double-blind, placebo-controlled trials, since they are used in the same way that orthodox medication is used.

The 'British Journal of Dermatology' reported that dermatologists at Great Ormond Street's Hospital for Sick Children used a Chinese remedy for eczema and found that the skin of most children in the trial improved by 60 per cent. Many of the remaining children improved when the remedy was individually adjusted for them. Japanese researchers found that a herbal prescription significantly reduced the chances of patients who suffered from cirrhosis subsequently developing liver cancer. Three new drugs are currently being developed from Chinese herbs in the United States, for use against malaria, Alzheimer's and HIV.

Researchers have found that the effects of many Chinese remedies are recognisable by practitioners of orthodox medicine, despite working from totally different concepts. Remedies for 'eliminating toxins' have an antiviral or antibacterial effect; those used to 'lower heat' do actually reduce fever and inflammation; 'tonics' stimulate the immune system, while other remedies aimed at treating 'stagnation' actually improve the circulation and have an anti-clotting effect.

In the same way, researchers have found that pressing the relevant points on the body does relieve pain and improve blood flow. Of course, they explain the results differently. They have found, for example, that the skin over acupressure points has a higher electrical conductivity than skin in the surrounding area. Stimulating these points causes the brain to release the natural pain-killing chemicals called endorphins. Tension in the surrounding muscles is relieved by pressure on the acupuncture point, allowing cramped blood vessels to expand and therefore to work more effectively.

Although far more research has been done on acupuncture (which is now widely accepted by doctors), acupressure has also made its mark in scientific trials. The acupressure point known as Pc 6 is probably the most renowned and frequently tested, having proved its ability to prevent nausea from a number of causes.

Acupressure fills an important gap in alleviating the nausea caused by pregnancy or by medicinal drugs, since nothing else does the job so well: pregnant women try to avoid taking medication, and although anti-emetic drugs can control vomiting, they do little to ease the horrible feeling of nausea.

Other research papers published in reputable journals extol the benefits of acupressure in looking after both the long-term ill and animals. It has been proved to treat infantile palsy, heart disease and respiratory ailments including asthma. It is also famous for relieving pain – most commonly headaches, muscular pain, angina, back ache and labour pains.

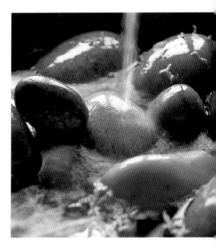

Reflexologists consider that all parts of the body are connected by subtle energy, which flows down the body from the head to the feet through 10 zones (sometimes called channels or vessels). When there is illness or discomfort the channels become blocked and the flow of energy is disturbed. Working on the hands and/or feet unblocks the channels, allows energy to flow and restores the balance, all of which relaxes the body, enhances the circulation and relieves the uncomfortable symptoms.

Relief can be almost immediate, but long-standing conditions may take some time to heal, since the healing begins on a deep level. Reflexologists believe the body heals itself from the inside to the outside. If symptoms have been suppressed by medical treatment they may return briefly in the order in which they were suppressed, which is why symptoms sometimes become worse for a while after the first few treatments.

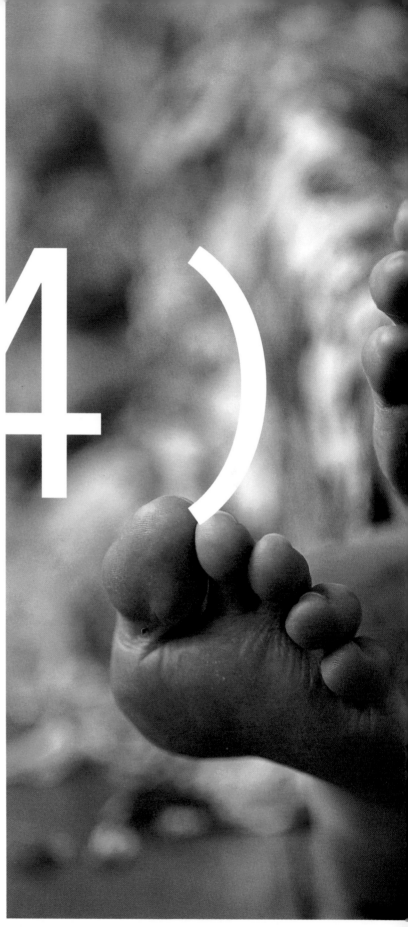

chapter four: reflexology

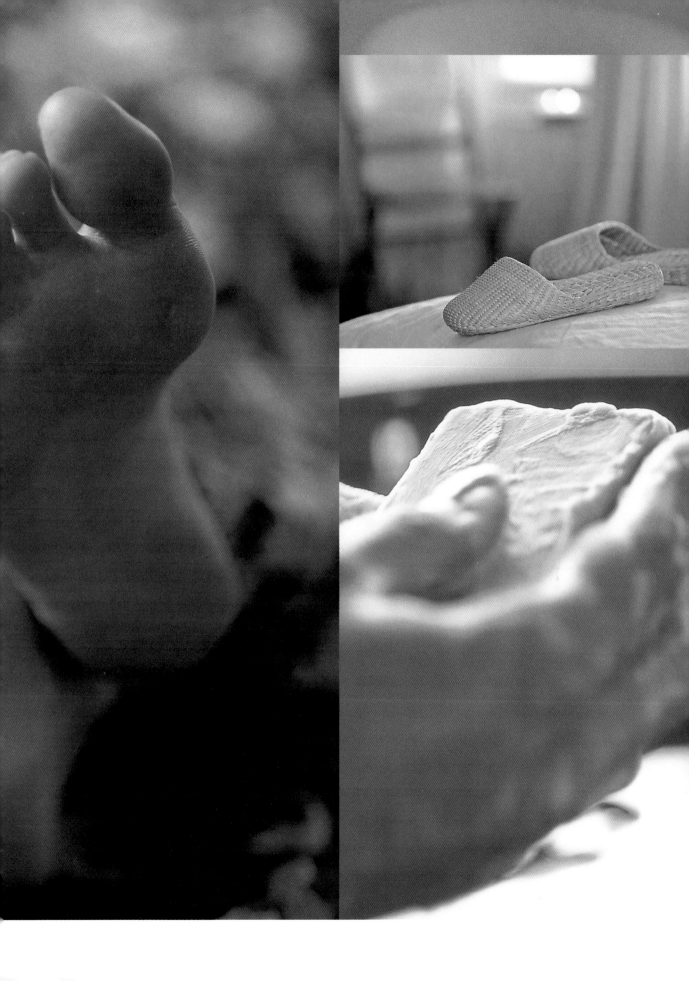

foot charts

The feet are extraordinary structures. Each of our feet contains 26 bones (together the feet hold a quarter of all the bones in our bodies), plus 7200 nerve endings and 107 ligaments. All of these structures provide exceptional strength and range of movement.

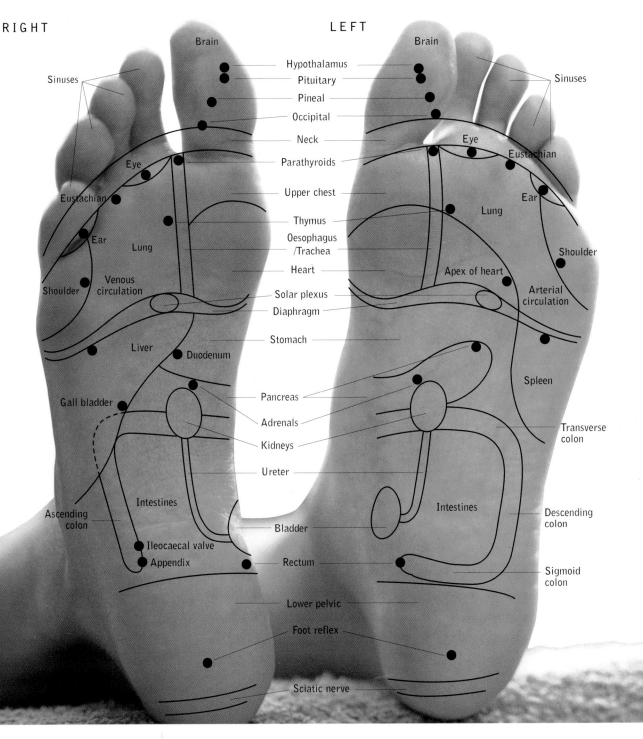

RIGHT

LEFT

Brain
Hypothalamus
Pituitary
Pineal
Occipital
Neck
Parathyroids
Upper chest
Thymus
Oesophagus /Trachea
Heart
Solar plexus
Diaphragm
Stomach
Duodenum
Pancreas
Adrenals
Kidneys
Ureter
Bladder
Rectum
Lower pelvic
Foot reflex
Sciatic nerve

Sinuses
Eye
Eustachian
Ear
Lung
Venous circulation
Shoulder
Liver
Gall bladder
Ascending colon
Intestines
Ileocaecal valve
Appendix

Brain
Sinuses
Eye
Eustachian
Ear
Lung
Shoulder
Apex of heart
Arterial circulation
Spleen
Transverse colon
Intestines
Descending colon
Sigmoid colon

In spite of being constantly trampled on, our feet are among the most sensitive parts of our bodies. For this reason the feet are the best place for reflexology treatments. Our hands, which we treat with a lot more respect, are actually much less sensitive than our feet.

Below and Left: **Notice that** some organs have particularly strong reflex points within their general area.

LEFT

RIGHT

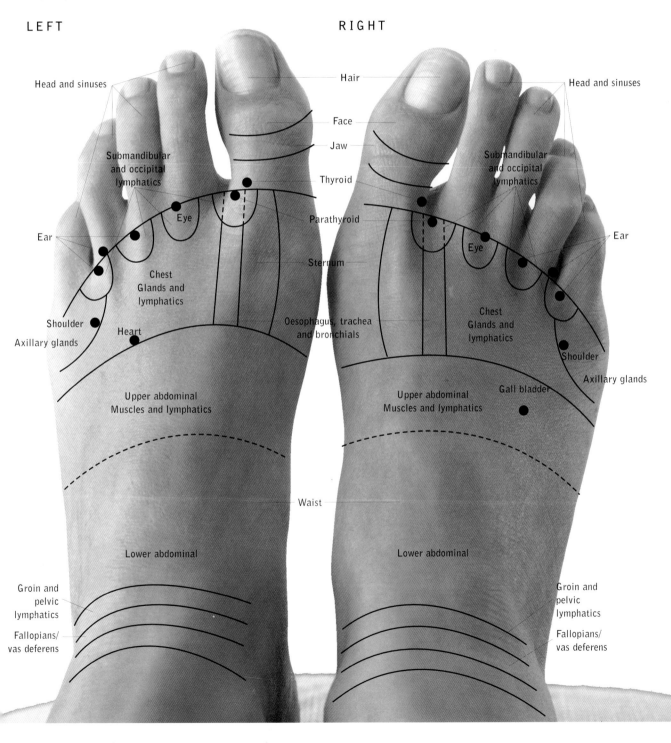

Head and sinuses

Hair

Submandibular and occipital lymphatics

Face

Jaw

Thyroid

Eye

Parathyroid

Ear

Sternum

Chest Glands and lymphatics

Shoulder

Oesophagus, trachea and bronchials

Axillary glands

Heart

Upper abdominal Muscles and lymphatics

Head and sinuses

Submandibular and occipital lymphatics

Eye

Ear

Chest Glands and lymphatics

Shoulder

Axillary glands

Gall bladder

Upper abdominal Muscles and lymphatics

Waist

Lower abdominal

Lower abdominal

Groin and pelvic lymphatics

Fallopians/ vas deferens

Groin and pelvic lymphatics

Fallopians/ vas deferens

how it works

Reflexology is a holistic complementary therapy. Its purpose is to treat the whole person, rather than a symptom, on the grounds that a symptom such as pain or a skin rash is usually the sign of an internal problem. Eliminating the symptom without solving the problem that caused it would be like trying to cure measles by painting over the spots. In addition, working exclusively on one part of the body may get the energy moving in that area, only to have it stagnate somewhere else. The patient may end up feeling worse rather than better. So a reflexologist normally starts by working on the entire foot in order to treat the entire person, before homing in on an area that requires extra help.

Whenever possible it is best to give both feet or hands a full treatment in this way. As well as restoring balance, it is also a soothing routine, whether you are working on yourself or someone else. Also, it is far more satisfying than leaving much of the foot or hand feeling neglected.

However, there are times when you don't have half an hour to do a full treatment, and others when a problem is just what it appears to be, rather than a sign of anything deeper – with travel sickness, for example. Even when there is a long-term inner problem, easing symptoms can be helpful while you do long-term work on its root cause.

A full reflexology treatment includes each of the system routines shown on the following pages, with the exception

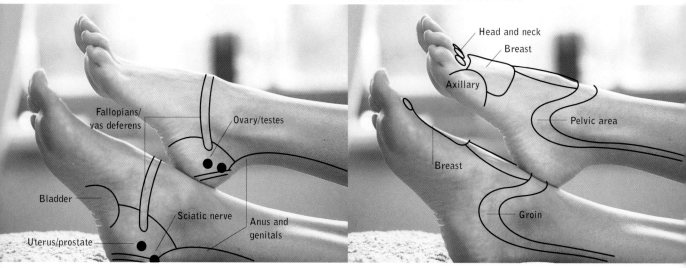

REPRODUCTIVE REFLEXES

Fallopians/
vas deferens
Ovary/testes
Bladder
Sciatic nerve
Anus and
genitals
Uterus/prostate

LYMPHATIC REFLEXES

Head and neck
Breast
Axillary
Pelvic area
Breast
Groin

of the endocrine (hormone) system, which is covered when you do all the others. This is shown separately so you can work on the entire endocrine system when you are dealing with a hormone-related problem. However, since there are endocrine glands in various parts of the body, you treat the entire endocrine system as you work your way through a full foot treatment.

If you do not have time to do a full treatment, start by awakening the energies using the brief preparatory sequence (see pages 40–45). Then just work on the system in which you have a problem before concentrating on individual points. For example, work the head and neck area for a headache followed by the specific head point.

Start and finish each section with long smooth strokes down the foot, stroking towards the ankle. Do the same after working on any sensitive areas, to ease discomfort and draw excess energy out of the area.

Anyone who has had a reflexology treatment should drink plenty of water afterwards. Reflexology enhances circulation and the nerve supply to all organs, so there is a balancing effect – which reflexologists call restoration of 'homeostasis', the body's equilibrium. Treatment may stimulate the body to release any stored toxins, which could cause headaches or nausea. Drinking plenty of water helps the kidneys work efficiently and flushes any waste products through and out of the body.

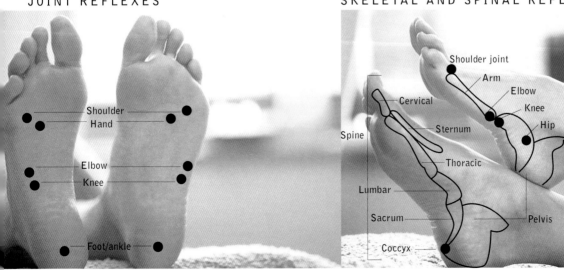

JOINT REFLEXES

Shoulder
Hand
Elbow
Knee
Foot/ankle

SKELETAL AND SPINAL REFLEXES

Shoulder joint
Arm
Elbow
Cervical
Knee
Spine
Sternum
Hip
Thoracic
Lumbar
Sacrum
Pelvis
Coccyx

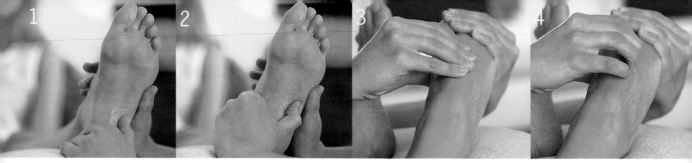

techniques

Most reflexology points are worked with the fingertips and the edge of the thumb, using firm pressure. You will probably use all the following methods during the course of one treatment on someone else. When working on your own foot, thumb- and finger-walking, rotation and flexing or pivoting on a point are the easiest methods.

Thumb- and finger-walking

Thumb-walking is carried out by flexing the thumb at the first joint while simultaneously sliding it forwards – similar to the movement of a caterpillar (see 1 and 2) . Finger-walking is carried out in the same way (see 3 and 4). The thumb or fingers never leave the skin, but their pressure fluctuates as they move.

Rotation on a point

Keep your thumb or index finger on one spot (5) and rotate it with slightly increased pressure in order to activate that point.

Pivoting on a point

Keep your supporting hand still and use your other hand to rotate the foot on your thumb or index finger while pressing into a point (6).

Flexing on a point

This is like pivoting, but instead of turning the foot you flex it towards the stationary thumb (7), gradually increasing and reducing the pressure.

Hook and back-up

Use this when you want to apply pressure to a special reflex point and when the point is deep within the foot and difficult to reach, or when you need to be very precise. Hold the foot so that the four fingers of the working hand are used as a lever and, with the outside edge of the thumb, press firmly on the point. Keep a steady pressure and – without moving the thumb from the point – draw the thumb backwards so that the tissue beneath it moves, while the thumb remains stationary. Hold for five seconds.

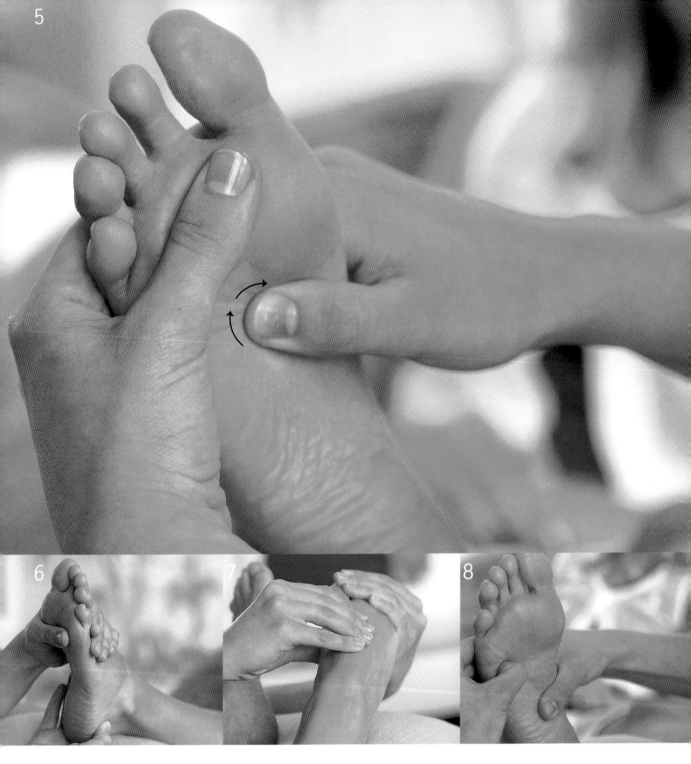

Hooking

The technique of hooking is sometimes used without the back-up when accessing a specific deep reflex such as the liver point or spleen point. In this case it is wise to hold for a count of five, then gradually release the pressure before moving the thumb (8). Hooking can be used to soothe a sensitive reflex.

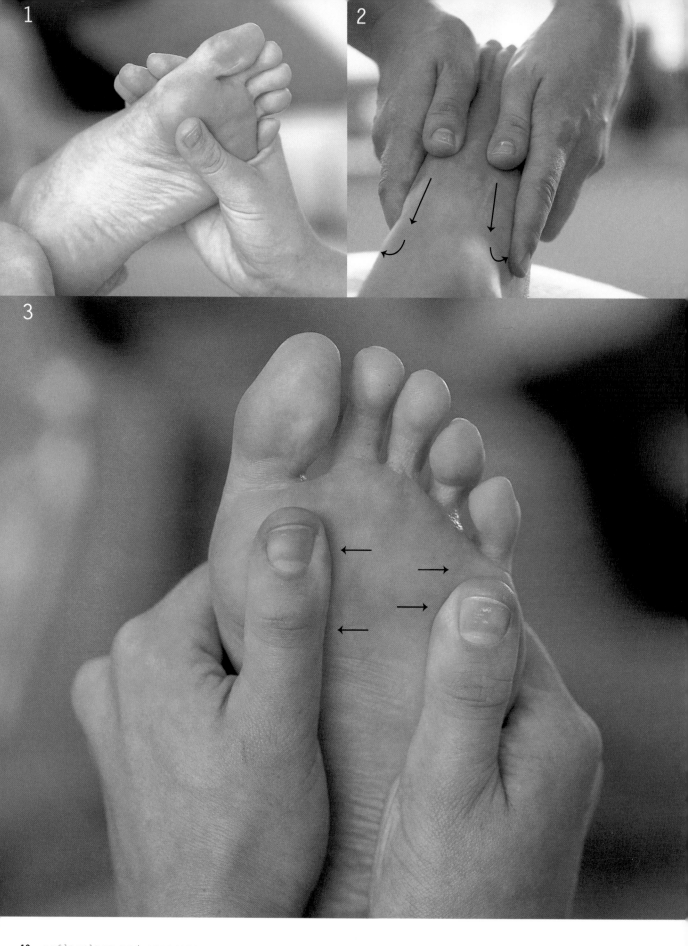

preparation

Your purpose is to relax the feet or hands you are working on and allow the energy to flow. Start by taking off your watch and any jewellery that may scratch the skin. Then cradle the foot in one hand – the supporting hand – while you work on it with the other – the working hand.

1 Holding the heel safely in one hand with the sole facing upwards and the other thumb on the instep, rotate the foot in both directions.

2 Then stroke firmly in both directions with both hands, down the foot from the toes to the ankles and back up to the toes.

3 Hold the foot in both hands and place the thumbs on the ball of the foot. Slide them out to the sides a few times, to create a feeling of openness.

4 Keeping your wrists loose and fingers slightly flexed, walk your thumb and fingers all over the feet or hands as shown, advancing in small steps without completely lifting the finger pads off the foot. Make sure you cover their full length and breadth. This movement arouses the energies in all five zones.

Whether you are working on yourself or someone else, make sure your finger movements are always walking forwards; in most cases it will be away from your body. This frees the energies and allows them to flow. When you are working on yourself you will soon get used to moving your hands and feet around to allow for this manoeuvre.

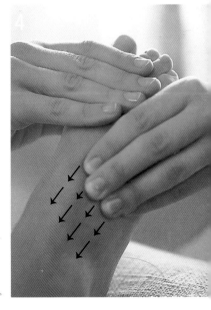

5 Thumb- and finger-walk each sole from the heel to the tips of the toes in five strips — one for each zone.

6 Work across the shoulder girdle located just below the base of the toes.

7 Next work across the diaphragm, located just below the ball of the foot.

8 Work across the pelvic floor, located just over the pad of the heel.

9 Finish these movements by thumb-walking several strips across the heel pad.

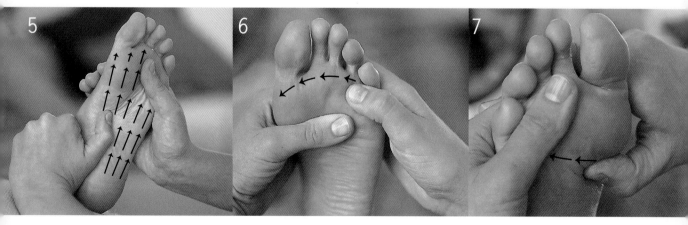

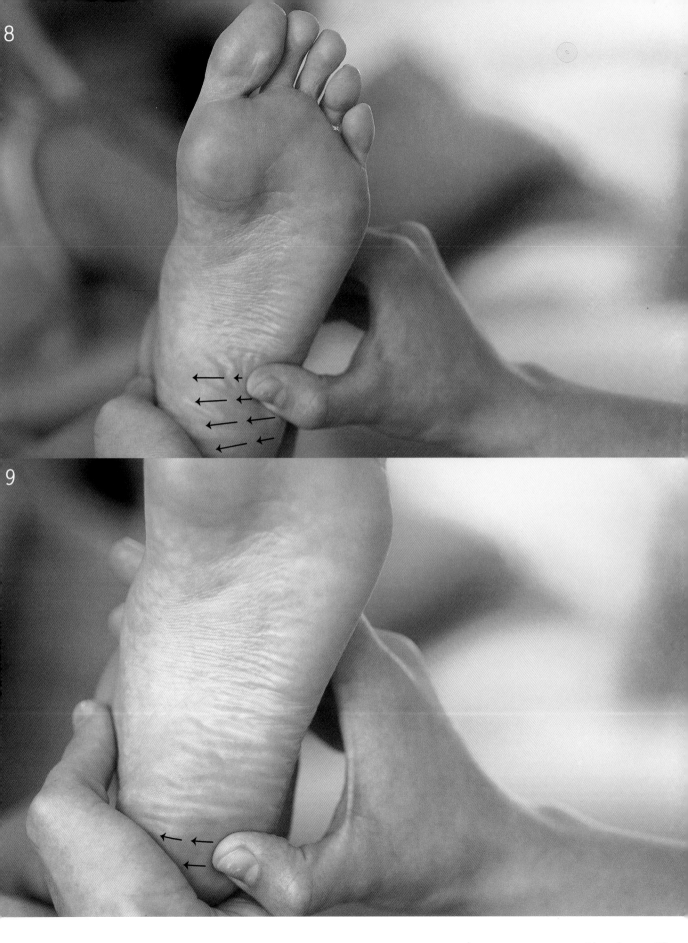

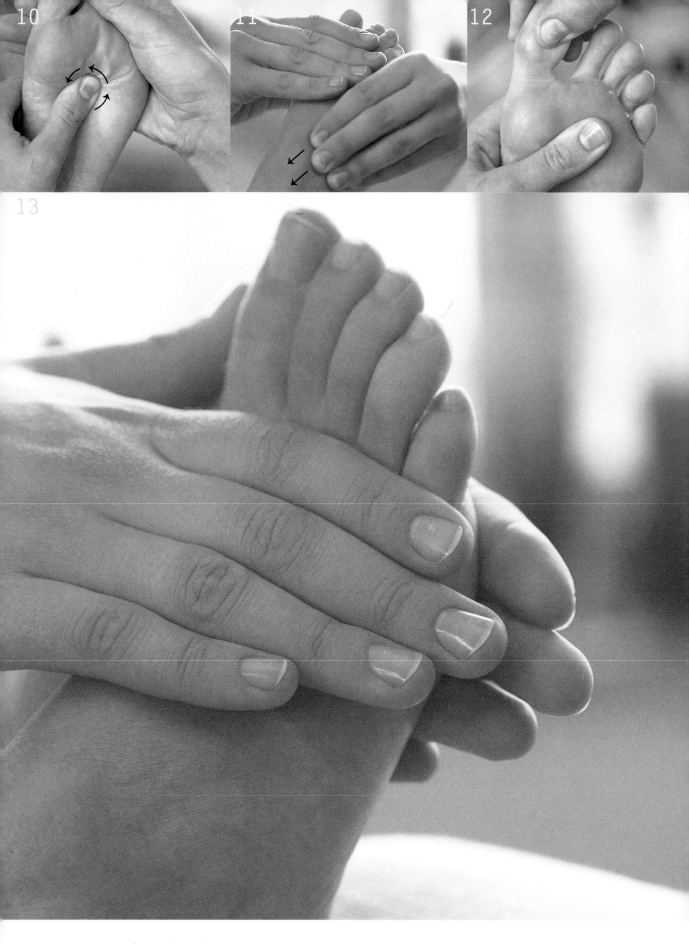

10 Next, cradling the foot in your hand, rotate your thumb in the solar plexus point. This is the spot in the centre of the foot from which the ball of the foot curves slightly down on each side – your thumb will slip into it quite naturally. Don't forget to add some long massage strokes along the length of the foot as you go along.

11 Turn the foot over if you are working on yourself. Walk your thumb and fingers diagonally across the top in both directions several times. Holding the foot comfortably, rotate the ankles to loosen them up.

12 Rotate each toe, and finish by pulling each one as if you were pulling a cap off it – firmly but without tugging.

13 Hold the foot between both palms, firmly enough to slide the skin over the bones, and rub the hands in circles. You can also do this using the back of the hand underneath the foot, if this feels comfortable.

14 Cradling the toes, thumb-walk all along the top of the ball of the foot just at the base of the toes, pressing firmly.

15 Massage the pads of the toes – the fleshy parts at the top of the underside – and then press your thumb into the tops of the toes, rotating the thumb. Work on both feet whenever possible, so you don't end up feeling off-balance.

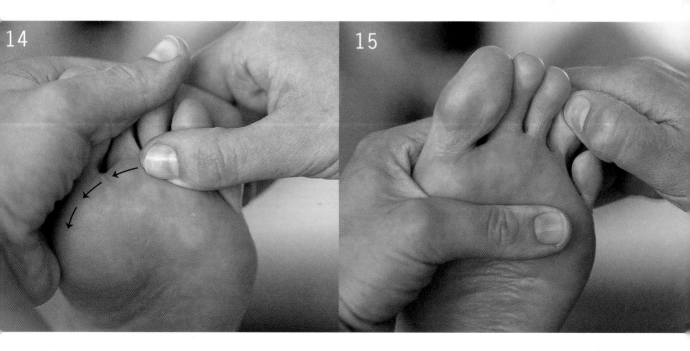

hand charts

Steps similar to those that apply to the feet apply to the hands. Walk your fingers or thumbs up the palms from the wrists to the tops of the fingers, making sure to cover each finger. Find the solar plexus point, similar to the one on the foot, and rotate the thumb on that while holding the hand in your other palm. Then work down the back, from the fingernails to the wrist, rotating the wrists and rotating and pulling each finger, as you did with the toes. Walk diagonally across, as you did on the feet.

To work on the systems of the hands, follow the same steps as you did on the feet, checking with the diagrams for details. The diagrams show both specific reflex points and more general organ areas for the right and left hands.

The only step you can't follow, if you are treating your own hand, is to hold it between both palms. In this case, rest your hand on a firm surface and rub in circles with the other hand.

Hand reflexology comes into its own in emergencies, when conditions don't allow time or space for working on the feet. It is also something you can do unobtrusively for yourself when you are out, for example to fend off travel sickness. For people who aren't used to physical therapies or feel self-conscious about their feet, a hand treatment offers many of the same benefits. Touch itself can be healing, and hand reflexology offers a very natural, acceptable way of providing a healing touch, using soothing massage-like techniques.

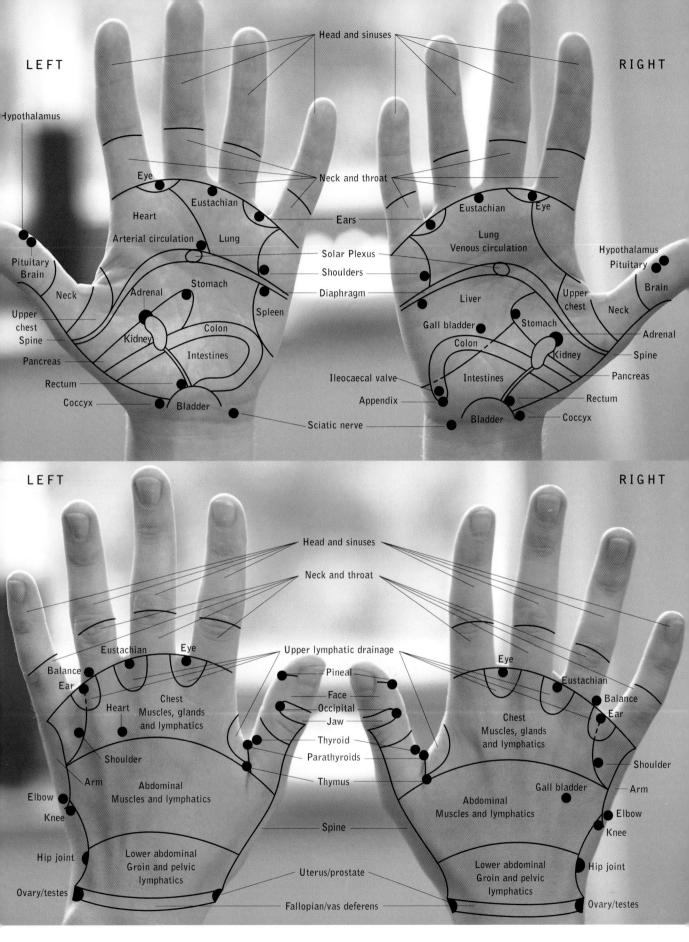

LEFT

RIGHT

Head and sinuses

Hypothalamus

Neck and throat

Eye

Eustachian

Heart

Ears

Eustachian

Eye

Arterial circulation

Lung

Solar Plexus

Lung
Venous circulation

Hypothalamus
Pituitary

Pituitary
Brain

Shoulders

Brain

Neck

Adrenal

Stomach

Diaphragm

Liver

Upper
chest

Neck

Upper
chest

Spleen

Gall bladder

Stomach

Adrenal

Spine

Kidney

Colon

Colon

Kidney

Spine

Pancreas

Intestines

Pancreas

Rectum

Ileocaecal valve

Intestines

Rectum

Coccyx

Bladder

Appendix

Coccyx

Sciatic nerve

Bladder

LEFT

RIGHT

Head and sinuses

Neck and throat

Eustachian

Eye

Upper lymphatic drainage

Eye

Balance
Ear

Pineal

Eustachian

Heart

Chest
Muscles, glands
and lymphatics

Face

Balance
Ear

Occipital
Jaw

Chest
Muscles, glands
and lymphatics

Shoulder

Thyroid

Shoulder

Arm

Parathyroids

Arm

Elbow

Abdominal
Muscles and lymphatics

Thymus

Gall bladder

Elbow

Knee

Abdominal
Muscles and lymphatics

Knee

Hip joint

Spine

Hip joint

Lower abdominal
Groin and pelvic
lymphatics

Uterus/prostate

Lower abdominal
Groin and pelvic
lymphatics

Ovary/testes

Fallopian/vas deferens

Ovary/testes

the reflex systems

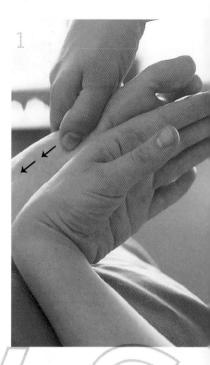

In reflexology the body is divided into 10 zones, numbered from one to five on each side of the body. The zones run from the tips of the toes to the head and back down to the fingertips, each one starting at a toe and at a finger or thumb and linking all parts of the body within one zone. Each zone one starts at the thumb and big toe, with the two zone fives starting at the little finger and the fifth toe on each side of the body. So zone three, for example, is the area starting at the middle toe or finger.

Reflexologists see the whole body reflected onto the hands or the feet, so most of the body is represented on each hand or foot. For this reason it is worth spending a bit of time working on each one. Double organs divide up in the obvious way, the right kidney or lung, for example, being represented on the right foot or hand. Other organs appear where you might expect: the heart point on the left foot or hand, since it is slightly left of centre in the chest, and the liver on the right. Most of the stomach is represented on the left foot but there is also a small stomach area on the right foot, mirroring its position in the abdomen and covering the pylorus and duodenum.

Reflexology is not an exact science and different charts may show slight differences in the location of organs and their points. This is because a practitioner's personal experience may lead to different conclusions, and because no two people are identical. Working over the meridians may also play a role. Charts are merely guides or route maps – one reason why it is best to work on the entire hand or foot.

You will notice that some organs are represented twice, with a small reflex point within a larger area bearing the same name – often the same shape as the organ reflected. This is because some organs have specific reflex points, which have been shown to stimulate or release tension within the organ even more than working on the whole organ area. A treatment generally includes pressing or hooking firmly on the specific reflex point for about five seconds, and also thumb- or finger-walking over the whole organ area.

ZONES AND SIDES

Draw four imaginary lines on your feet, starting between the toes and slicing on down through the heels. Zone one is the strip containing your big toe, zone two the second toe and so on. The little toe is in zone five.

Throughout this book you will read about the 'inside' and the 'outside' of the foot. Imagine your footprint: the inside is the edge from the big toe to the heel and the outside is from the little toe to the outside of the heel. The same applies to the hands: the inside is nearest the thumb, the outside nearest the little finger.

Incidentally, remember that the bones of the toe start farther down the foot than we can see; flex your toes to feel the joint between the toes and the foot bones about a thumb-width down.

WORKING FORWARDS

Always work forwards, away from yourself (1). Reflexology is meant to facilitate the flow of energy to remove blockages: working back towards yourself is less effective, and you may even deplete your own energy. It is rather like using a hosepipe to clear a drain – aim it away from yourself. Keep changing position or turning the hand or foot in order to avoid working back towards yourself.

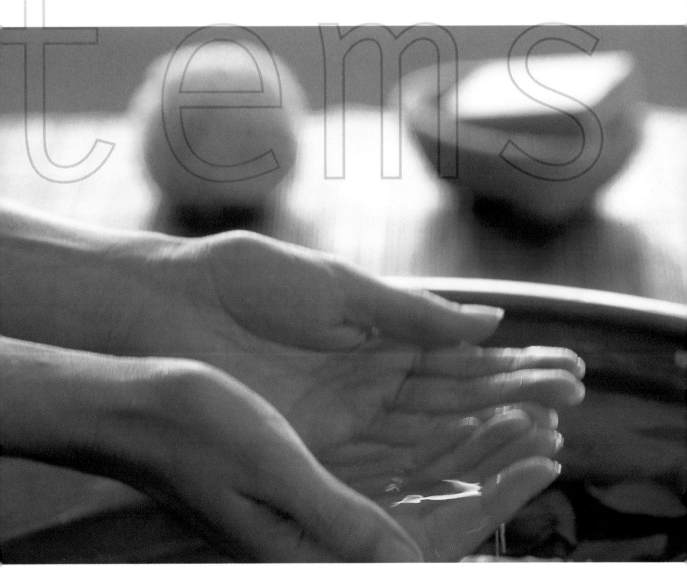

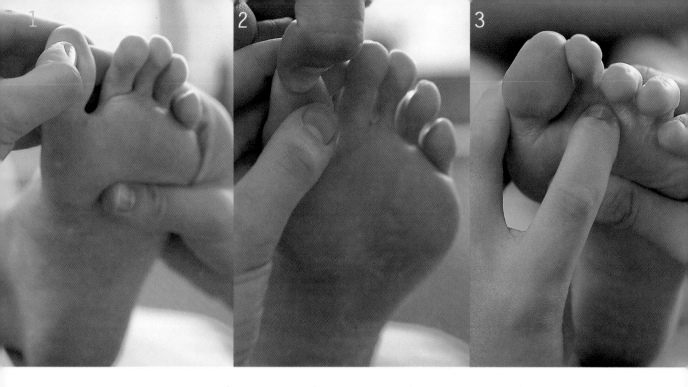

head and neck area

The brain and central nervous system are centred on the big toe. Covering all the toes will work these, plus the face and the glands, muscles and sensory organs in that area. Work this system to treat disorders such as headache, migraine, insomnia, stress, sciatica, tinnitus, sensory problems (eyes, ears and nose), multiple sclerosis and epilepsy.

Start by walking your thumb up the pad of the big toe several times, until you have covered the whole expanse. Then walk your index finger down the front and sides in the same way. Remember you are always moving away from your body.

The nail represents your face and hair and the sides are the big muscles up the sides of your neck, so work carefully on these if you have problems in the area, still thumb- and finger-walking. Don't spend too long on any one area — you don't want to overstimulate it. Walk across the back of the big toe to free up neck muscles. Work across the sides and front of the big toe below the nail with the index finger for the teeth, jaw and throat.

The pituitary gland — the master gland, controlling the hormone production of all other glands — is situated in the brain, and represented by a spot in the exact centre of the big toe pad. Hold the foot in the supporting hand, with the fingers behind the big toe, and hook into the pituitary point with the thumb of the working hand, using four-finger leverage against the supporting hand (1). Remember: don't pinch.

After five seconds, use the opposite thumb to press into another important gland, the hypothalamus, on top of the toe just above the pituitary (2). If this is a little difficult, simply press and rotate, covering both points.

On the top of the foot at the base of the big toe is the thyroid point. Using your index finger, hook in and press for five seconds. Next, to stimulate the parathyroids in the web between the big toe and second toe, pinch gently but firmly into the web and hold for a count of five.

Slide diagonally down from the centre of the big toe pad to the corner of the pad beside the next toe. This is the occipital spot, representing the bony ridge of the back of your skull. It is a good place to massage if you have tension headaches or neck pain.

Drawing an imaginary line between the pituitary and the occipital – from the centre of the big toe pad to the lower corner beside the next toe – find a spot halfway between the two, which represents the pineal gland. The pineal gland regulates your body clock and helps you sleep. Work on these points with firm thumb pressure by hooking in and holding an even pressure for five seconds.

For the eye (left eye on the left foot, right eye on the right), press into the fleshy area between and just below the bottom of the second and third toes, supporting with the other hand (3). Press and hold this for three to five seconds, or press and release if it is too sensitive. Do the same for the ear; press down into the fleshy part between and just below the fourth and the fifth toe.

Finger walk up and down the front, back and sides of all the toes except the big toe. This helps sinus drainage to the upper lymphatics, the glands in the neck area.

Turning the foot over to work on the top, press the balance point at the bottom of the fourth toe just next to the fifth toe (4). Complete the session by stroking the foot.

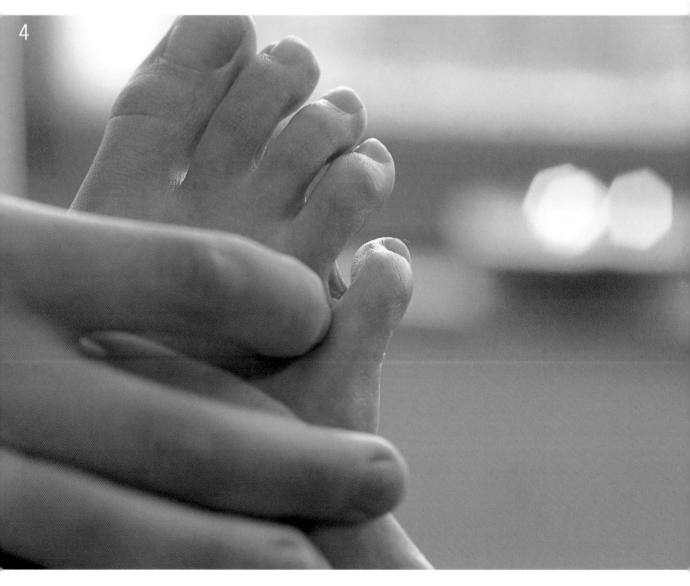

4

chest area

Stretching across the ball of each foot is an area that includes both the respiratory system (asthma, bronchitis, emphysema, hay fever and allergic reactions) and the cardio-vascular system (disorders of the heart and circulation, including angina, high blood pressure, varicose veins and cold fingers).

Cradling your foot in one hand, draw an imaginary line down the ball of the foot from a point between the big and second toes. This represents the oesophagus and trachea. Walk down this line and up again with your thumbs, finishing by resting the thumb of your cradling hand on that line. Then walk the other thumb horizontally from the bony edge of the foot across the ball of the foot under the big toe, covering zone one (see 1). This works on the nerves that supply the heart, lungs and the chest area.

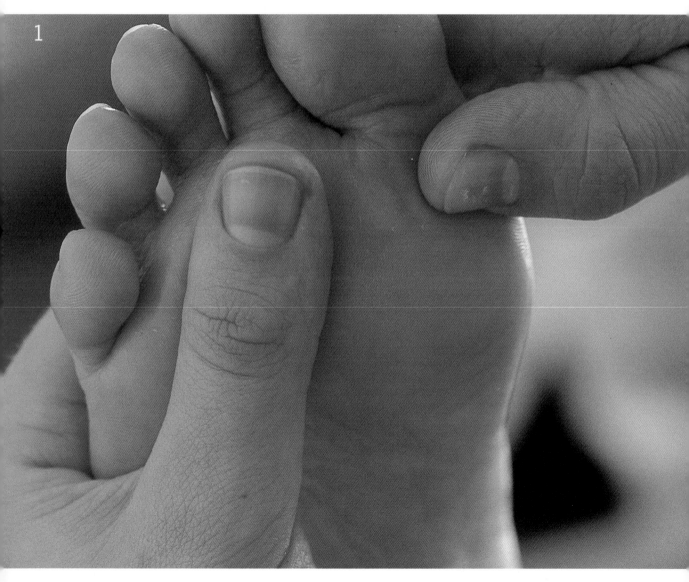

1

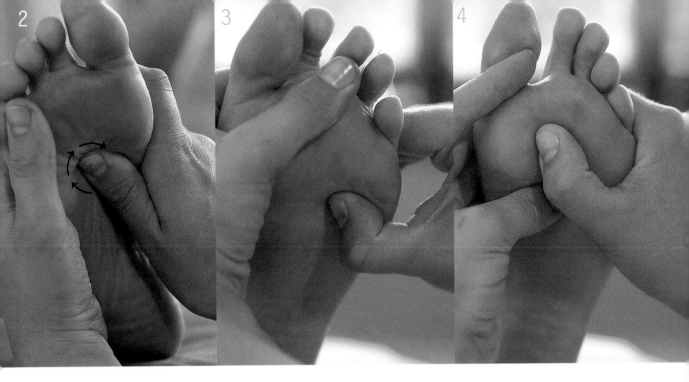

If possible, change hands to keep the flow of energy going in the right direction. Finding the bottom of the ball of the foot, thumb-walk its entire length to help relax the diaphragm. Change hands again and work back. You will notice how the ball of the foot curves up near the centre and then down, as if it is made in two sections.

Next rotate the thumb and massage the centre point (2), which is the solar plexus. The diaphragm and the solar plexus are important areas, particularly for any problem that is stress-related.

Change hands (to ensure that you are still working away from your body) and thumb-walk back, this time across the ball of the foot itself, to stimulate the circulation – veins on the right foot and arteries on the left. Walk horizontally across several times, from the outside edge (under the little toe) to the inside edge, to cover the whole ball of the foot.

To work the bronchi (the tubes in the lungs that go into spasm during an asthma attack), walk your thumb up from the bottom of the ball of the foot vertically, in zone two. Work in several strips to cover the whole area, and continue into zones two and three to work the lungs (zone five is the arm and shoulder area).

On the left foot, thumb-walk across zones two to four on the ball of the foot to nourish the heart. Find the heart point at the base of the fourth toe joint, at the lower edge of the ball of the foot, and press upwards towards the fifth toe, with your thumb on the sole next to the diaphragm and your index finger on the other side of your foot for a pinching effect (3). Hold firmly for five seconds to ease the tension, releasing gently if the point is sensitive.

The thymus gland is halfway down the oesophagus line on the ball of the foot. Cradling the inside of the foot, hook in on the point towards the bone of the big toe and gently back up (4). Hold for five seconds.

On the top of the foot, the breasts are represented by an area about 25mm (1in) deep just below the toes and covering most of the width of the foot. Walk horizontal strips with all four fingers across this area. Overlap each row to cover the whole armpit and breast area.

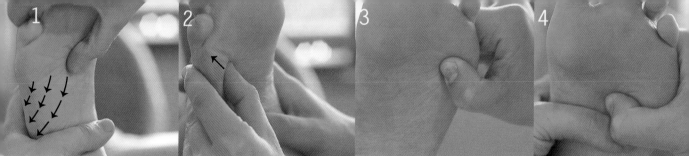

abdomen, digestive and eliminatory systems

This covers the area across each sole below the ball of the foot, as well as most of the instep below that. Many of the vital organs are represented in this area, including most of the digestive system, so you can cover most of the organs quite simply by working back and forth across both feet. If you divide the instep in half at its highest point, this will give you the approximate position of the waistline, which is a good landmark for locating the individual organs. To be specific you can work the following.

For the liver, work diagonally in both directions on the right foot, covering the large area indicated in a triangular shape, starting at the edge of the diaphragm next to the oesophagus and going right down to the small protrusion (the elbow point) on the outside edge of the foot (1). The specific liver point is located below the diaphragm and is worked by hooking and applying firm pressure towards the fifth toe (2).

The spleen is in a similar area on the left foot but only covers zones three, four and five. The spleen point is also found beneath the diaphragm (3) and can be worked by hooking towards the fifth toe.

The stomach is found mainly on the left foot, although part of it is on the right, together with the duodenum and pylorus. Work these by walking and rotating down the centre of the right foot on a line roughly between zones two and three. Work over the stomach in horizontal strips on both feet.

The pancreas lies below the stomach. Its specific point can be located on the left foot (4), in the third zone just below the stomach, a little above the waistline.

The gall bladder has its own specific point on the right foot, and can be accessed by pinching gently through the foot, with the index finger on top of the foot beneath the fourth toe, and the thumb hooked under the third toe a little above the waistline (5). Working back and forth diagonally, remember to turn your foot (or change position if you are treating someone else) when necessary in order to keep the movement out and away from your body.

Next, thumb-walk very thoroughly up, down and across the small intestine area, a strip about 25mm (1in) deep stretching the whole width of the instep just above the heel and below the waistline on both feet. This covers metres of intestine and should be worked thoroughly.

To work the colon on the right foot, start in zone four just above the heel. Apply pressure firmly for about five seconds on both the ileocaecal valve and the appendix, then thumb-walk up towards the waistline. You need to follow the route of this organ – first the ascending colon (6), towards the waistline, and then across part of the transverse colon (7), working horizontally to the inside edge of the foot.

At this stage you can choose whether to change feet or continue on the right foot. Some people prefer to work the whole colon in one go. If you want to do so, you have to change feet now, since the colon crosses the whole body. Press the inside edges of the feet together and, starting in zone one on the left foot, continue to thumb-walk across the foot to zone five.

Having walked across the foot, change hands so you can walk downwards towards the heel on the descending colon (8). Change direction again just before the heel pad, walking back along the sigmoid colon (9) towards the inner edge of the foot.

Finally, rotate your inside thumb, pressing it into the rectum point (10) on the inside edge of the heel pads to finish. Cover the pelvic floor and buttock muscles by walking across the heel pads. If you don't want to change feet, just slot the second half of the colon in after the intestines on the left foot sequence.

CHANGING DIRECTIONS

Unless you are very acrobatic, you will have to change your foot position along the way – particularly if you are working on yourself – to keep the movement going away from your body. Working on someone else, you will have to change hands as needed so that you are comfortable. Remember to keep your support hand actively engaged at all times as you work.

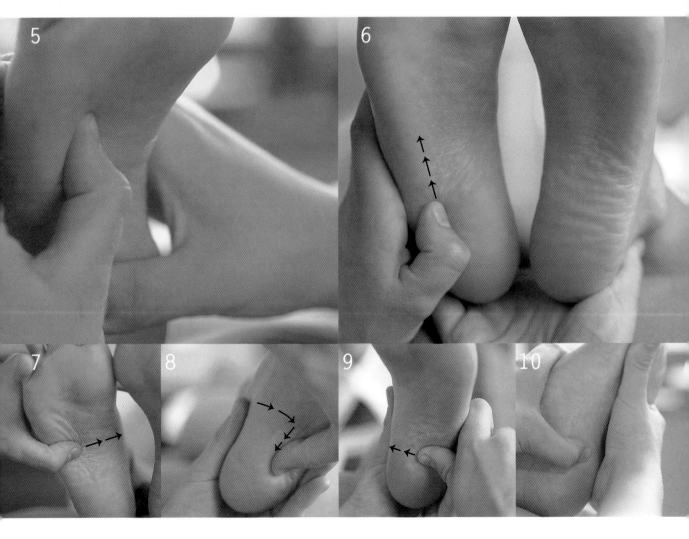

urinary and reproductive systems

The bladder is easy to find. It is a slightly puffy area about the size of a 10 pence piece on the inside edge of the foot, just above the heel (1). Thumb-walk several times over the bladder area, fanning out to cover it all. Then, starting from the centre of the bladder, walk slightly towards the centre of the foot (you will feel the extensor tendon), turn your thumb to face the toes and walk up the ureter (2) towards the kidneys. Keep holding the foot firmly with your support hand.

The kidneys are found in zone two, level with the waistline. The adrenal glands are just above the kidneys, slightly behind them on the edge of zone one and rather difficult to reach. Press and hold firmly on the kidney area as your working thumb reaches it, pointing towards the toes. With your other thumb pointing down the foot, quickly press into the adrenal point (3) while simultaneously releasing the pressure of the first thumb on the kidney. This area is often sensitive, so ease excess energy out of the area afterwards by stroking firmly down towards the heel.

For the reproductive organs, work over the side of your foot, in an area between the back of the heel and the ankle bone. Gently walk all four fingers up to the ankle bone, covering the soft area that takes up the width of the heel. If working on yourself, turn your foot to make sure you are still working forwards. Find the uterus or prostate point

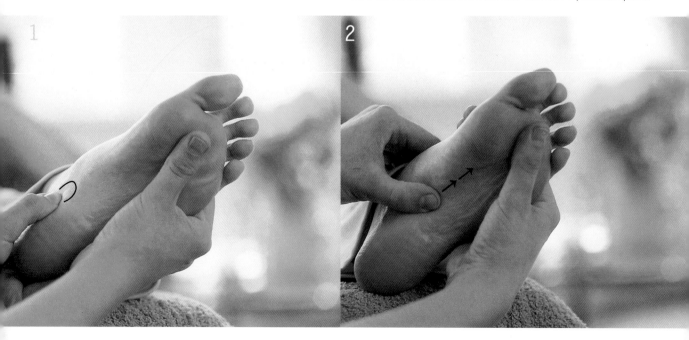

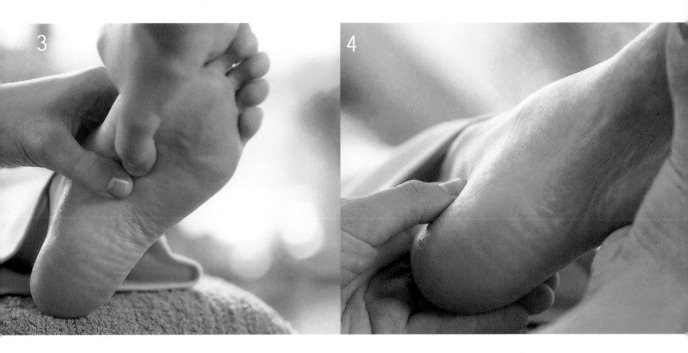

midway between the ankle bone and the tip of the heel (4). Holding the tip of the foot in the other hand, press this spot firmly with your thumb. You can then use your supporting hand to rotate the foot towards your thumb pressure. In this way you can increase and decrease the pressure to this sensitive point as needed.

Women's fallopian tubes and men's vas deferens cover a thin strip across the top of the foot, like an ankle strap, linking the uterus/prostate point on the inside of the foot with the matching ovary/testis point at the same spot on the outside. Using two fingers, walk its length from the uterus/prostate point. Finish by massaging the ovary/testis point with your thumb for a moment before firmly pressing.

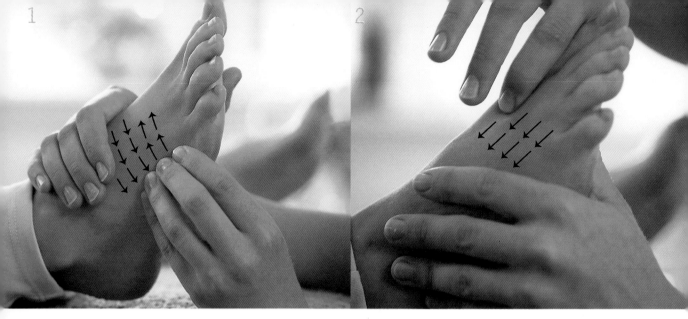

lymphatic system

The lymphatic system drains wastes from the body's cells
with the help of lymph nodes which are situated
throughout the body, with large collections in the chest,
groin and armpits. Good lymphatic drainage is essential to
help the body cleanse itself.

Starting from the ankle, walk firmly around the soft
areas on both sides of the ankle, feeling into all the little
bony crevices, using all four fingers and overlapping the
fallopian tubes and vas deferens. This will ensure you
cover all the lymph nodes in the groin area.

Move to the top edge of the bony ridge of zone one (1)
and walk horizontal strips with all four fingers,
overlapping slightly to cover the whole of the foot. Finish
on the top of the foot beneath the toes. This will cover the
lymph nodes of the abdomen, breast and armpit.
Although you have already worked these while covering
the chest area, it is well worth giving this important
system some extra attention.

To improve lymphatic drainage, walk your index finger
down between the toes towards the instep, then gently
draw it back towards the toes (2). To complete the
drainage, gently 'milk' the lymph nodes by rotating the
thumb and index finger on both sides of the foot at the
base of the toes.

endocrine system: the hormones

This system is mainly used when you are working on hormonal problems without doing a full treatment. Start by working the master gland, the pituitary, then the hypothalamus, which connects with the nervous system. Cradling the foot, hook into the pituitary point with the working thumb, in the exact centre of the big toe pad, for a count of five, making sure you don't pinch. Then press with the other thumb into the hypothalamus, on top of the toe just above the pituitary. If this is difficult, just press and rotate on both points.

The thyroid is located on the top of the foot at the base of the big toe (1). Using your index finger, hook in and press this point for five seconds. Next, to stimulate the parathyroids in the web between the big toe and second toe (2), pinch gently but firmly into the web and hold for a count of five.

The thymus is important, particularly if there is an infection producing mucus. First find the thymus halfway down the oesophagus on the ball of the foot, then, cradling the inside of the foot, hook in on the point towards the bone of the big toe and continue with a gentle back-up movement. Hold for five seconds.

The adrenal glands are just above the waistline on the edge of zone one. To work them, press and hold firmly on the kidney area (slightly below in zone one, level with the waistline) and, with your other thumb pointing down the foot, quickly press into the adrenal point while releasing pressure on the kidney. This is often a tender spot, so stroke firmly down towards the heel afterwards.

Next work over the spleen, finishing by hooking in towards the fifth toe for five seconds. It is important to work both the spleen and thymus in order to boost the immune system.

The biggest gland in the body is the pancreas, which is important for balancing blood sugar. There is a pancreas area on both feet, but the reflex point is found on the left foot, just a little above the waist in the centre of the foot. Hook and hold on this point for five seconds.

Find the ovary/testis point midway between the ankle bone and the tip of the heel on the outside of the foot. Massage it with your thumb before firmly pressing for a count of five.

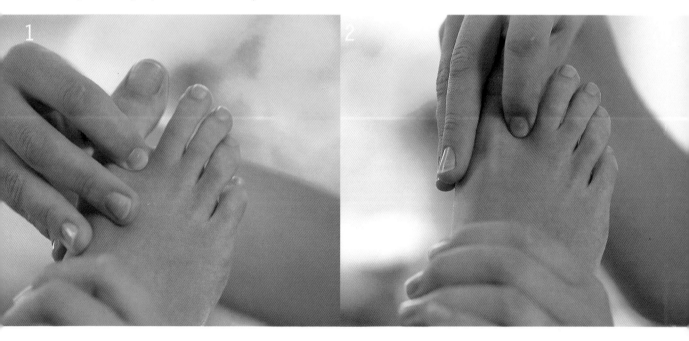

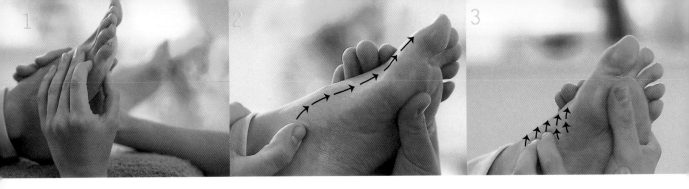

skeleton and muscles

This helps spinal problems, shoulders, neck, repetitive stress injury (RSI), carpal tunnel syndrome, arthritis and rheumatism, among others.

Pinch the shoulder point (1) between the fourth and fifth toe joints (about a finger-width below the toe). Lift and rotate all the toes – representing the sides of the neck – and flex the ball of the foot in order to relieve any stiffness that is present in the ribs.

The spinal reflexes run the full length of the inside of the foot, from the neck at the side of the big toe to the coccyx at the corner of the heel bone (2). Thumb walk up the side of the foot from the heel to the bony swelling at the base of the big toe joint, then continue along the edge of the big toe to the base of the big toe pad to cover the neck – the cervical bone reflexes. If you are working on yourself, turn the foot so you are still working forwards and away from yourself (although your thumb will now be pointing back towards your body) and walk down to the heel again. Complete the spinal reflexes by working in small horizontal strips across the spinal muscles (3).

Using all four fingers, cross the bony inside edge of the foot. Work all the way from the heel to the base of the big toe. Finish with massage strokes down the inside edge of the foot, toe to heel, to clear the energy field.

To complete the skeletal reflexes, pinch gently but firmly through the shoulder reflex, on the foot between the fourth and fifth toe bones, about a finger-width below the toes. It is down where the toe bones meet the foot bones – flex your toes up and down to find the spot.

Next work with your index finger down the bony outer edge of the foot, covering the arm to the elbow. The small bony protrusion half way down is the elbow point (4). Press on this for five seconds, releasing gradually.

The knee reflex (5) is beneath the elbow reflex. With the tip of your thumb, press in under the elbow point and draw firmly towards the small toe, holding for five seconds.

The hip reflex (6) and thigh are a little difficult to reach if you are working on yourself, but make sure you have worked well around the bony heel, particularly the outside edge. Support the heel in the palm of one hand and find a small bony protuberance about 25mm (1in) below the ankle bone with the middle finger of the working hand. Using your index finger, draw back towards the ankle bone and hold the pressure on the hip joint for a count of five.

The sciatic points (7) are behind the heel, on the top of the heel bone, just off the Achilles tendon. Gently rotate your thumb or finger on them.

The foot has a reflex of its own, found in the centre of the heel pad. Again, rotate and press on this with your thumb. The hand point (8) is just below the diaphragm between zones three and four. Rotate your thumb and press on this area. This is often an area of great tension, perhaps because when we are stressed we are mentally clenching our fists. Working this area and the spinal reflexes can be highly effective in releasing pressure and tension from the chest. This in turn enhances breathing and circulation, helping to ward off further tension.

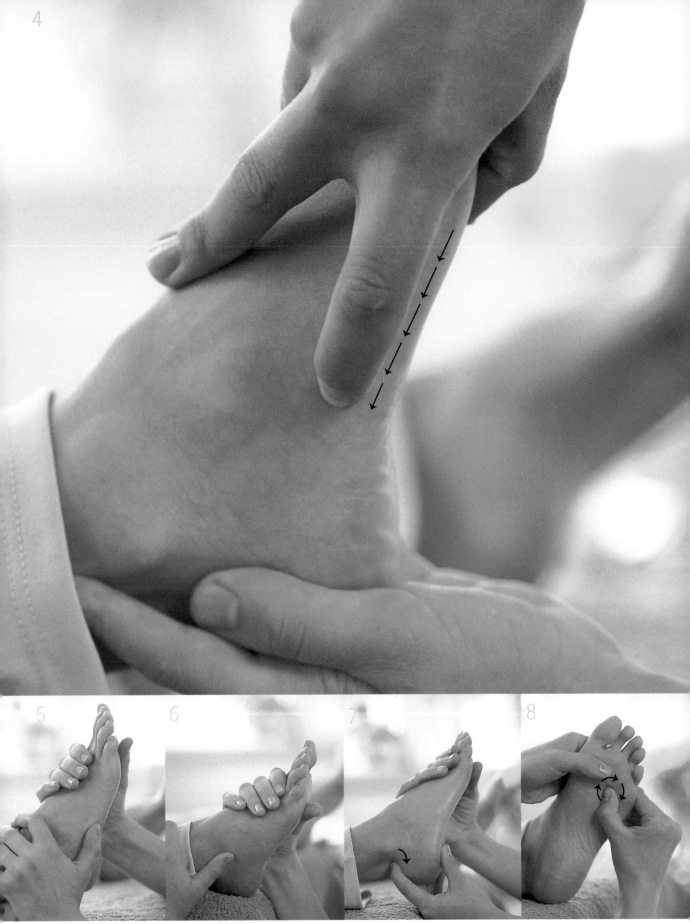

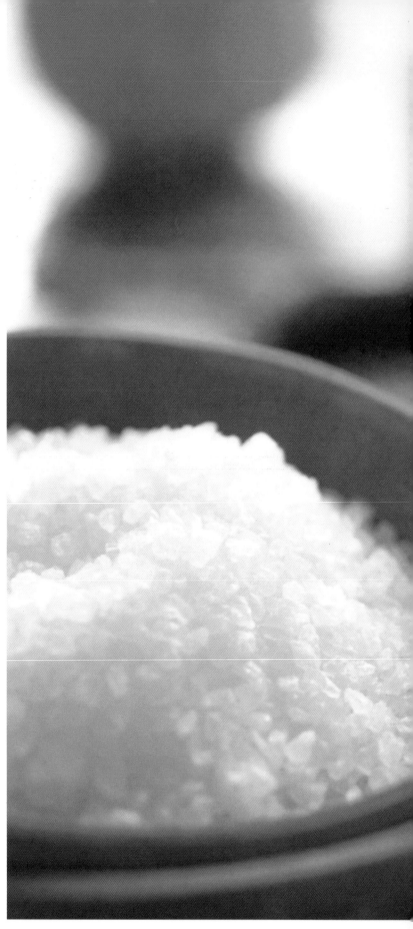

Like reflexology, acupressure works on one area in order to affect another. Although it follows a different map – the ancient Chinese meridians rather than the more recent concept of zones – most of the principles are similar.

Over the centuries the Chinese body map has developed into a vast and complex structure working on a number of levels, including the spiritual. As well as the meridians named in this book, there are also 15 'collaterals' that connect the organ meridians (rather like the escalators between underground railway lines) and eight extra meridians that store energy.

However, this book is meant for simple home treatment, so we are not concerned with the sort of detail that acupuncturists have to master. Of the 22 meridians and 660 pressure points, we will only be using the most valuable and those that are easy to find. The analogy is more appropriate to a first aid and self-help course than to a medical degree.

chapter five: acupressure

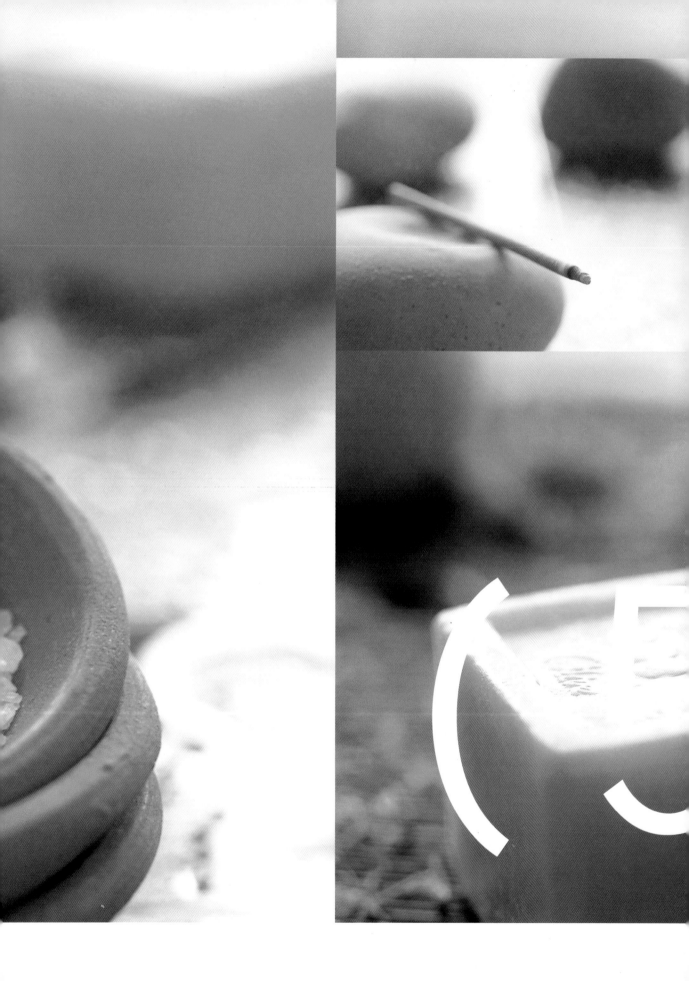

the meridians

There are 14 main meridians, six on each side of the body and one each down the centre of the front and the back. Twelve of these are each connected to one of the internal organs and have a greater effect on that organ.

The meridians are grouped in pairs: one yin and one yang. Yin energy comes from the Earth, so meridians carrying more yin energy start from the lowest point: the first point on the spleen meridian, for example, is on the big toe. Yang meridians are numbered from the top, since they receive yang energy from the Sun: the bladder meridian, for example, starts beside the eye. There are two of each of the organ meridians. They follow identical pathways on the left and the right side of the body. The other two meridians we will be using are called the governor vessel, which runs up the spine and over the head, and the conception vessel, which runs up the centre front of the body.

Stroking or massaging your skin along the route of a meridian is said to help balance the body's systems. And particular points on the meridian are especially beneficial to work on. There are literally hundreds of these acupressure points; this book includes some of the most valuable and easiest to work on without professional knowledge, and mentions just some of their attributes. The points you need to work on are often quite easy to find when you move your fingers sensitively over the skin, for example in a natural dip.

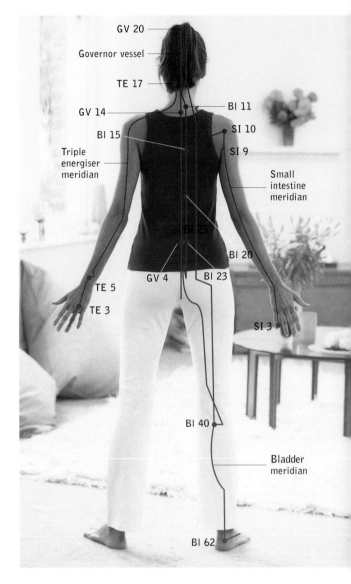

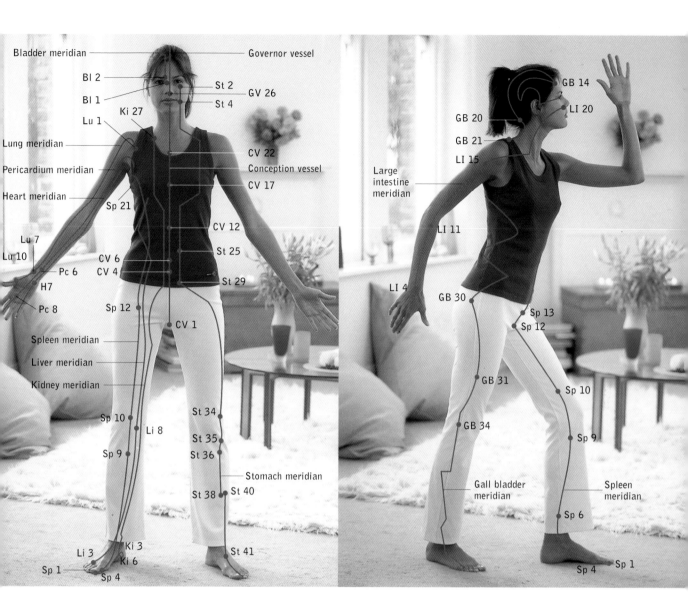

Bladder meridian
Governor vessel
Bl 2
St 2
GV 26
Bl 1
St 4
Ki 27
Lu 1
Lung meridian
CV 22
Pericardium meridian
Conception vessel
CV 17
Heart meridian
Sp 21
CV 12
St 25
Lu 7
CV 6
Lu 10
CV 4
St 29
Pc 6
H7
Pc 8
Sp 12
Spleen meridian
CV 1
Liver meridian
Kidney meridian
Sp 10
St 34
Li 8
St 35
Sp 9
St 36
Stomach meridian
St 38
St 40
Li 3
Ki 3
St 41
Ki 6
Sp 1
Sp 4

GB 14
GB 20
LI 20
GB 21
LI 15
Large intestine meridian
LI 11
LI 4
GB 30
Sp 13
Sp 12
GB 31
Sp 10
GB 34
Sp 9
Gall bladder meridian
Spleen meridian
Sp 6
Sp 4
Sp 1

OTHER POINTS

Not all acupressure points are on a meridian. A whole series of other points also affect the body's energy flow – those on the ears that treat high blood pressure, for example – and do not have a number.

Trigger points are different again. These are tender spots, where acupressure overlaps with anatomy. The trigger points are full of nerve endings. The value of a trigger point is that it connects with the source of the pain. With sciatica, for example, a trigger point on the leg will be tender, but working on it can relieve pain that is coming from where the nerve begins, in the base of the spine. There are several trigger points on the calves, which trigger release of muscle pain and cramp.

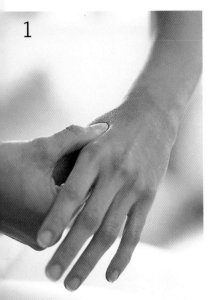

LUNG MERIDIAN

The lung meridian runs from the top of the chest down to the thumb. As well as their physical aspect, in Chinese philosophy the points situated here are linked with tears and sorrow.

Lung 1: between the first and second ribs, about a hand-width out from the breastbone; for respiratory diseases such as bronchitis and emphysema.

Lung 7: put the webbing between thumb and forefinger of one hand against the same area on the other and clasp your hands so your top index finger stretches down the wrist of the lower hand. Lung 7 is the point your index finger reaches on the bone below the side of the thumb.

Lung 10: on the pad of the thumb two finger-widths from the wrist, right on the edge of the thumb bone. Lung 7 and 10 are good points for releasing stagnation, allowing blocked energy to move and freeing any repressed emotions.

LARGE INTESTINE MERIDIAN

This runs upwards, from the index finger to the edge of the nose. It is responsible for cleansing and detoxifying.

LI 4: between finger and thumb. Press your thumb against the first finger and see where the webbing bulges up highest. Put your other thumb on that point, then – letting the first thumb open out away from the hand – hold that point with finger and thumb. This is called the great eliminator (1), excellent for constipation and getting things moving.

Warning: this point must not be used during pregnancy.

LI 11: with your arm folded across your chest, press into the end of the fold on top of the elbow joint. Eases arthritic pain, especially in the shoulder.

LI 20: run your fingers down the side of the nose and press into the wing at the bottom outer edge of the nostril. This is good for treating sinusitis and upper respiratory tract infections.

STOMACH MERIDIAN

The stomach meridian is associated with balancing and nourishing the system. It runs down the body from the head to the second toe.

St 2: middle of bone directly below eye. For eyesight and for releasing tension from the face.

St 4: corner of the mouth when mouth is at rest. For relaxing the facial muscles: useful in cases of extreme tension, toothache or Bell's palsy.

St 25: two thumb-widths beside the navel. For constipation, diarrhoea and indigestion.

St 29: a hand-width below the navel, two thumb-widths out. Women's problems, including problems with the ovaries, and premenstrual syndrome (PMS).

St 34: two thumb-widths above the knee, from the outer edge of the knee cap.

St 35: bottom of the knee cap, one each side of the centre.

St 36: find a bump just below your kneecap, towards the outside of the leg. Measure three finger-widths down the bone and press. Called the 'three-mile point' (2), this is what's known as a 'sea point' – the spot where it is easiest to access the energy of an entire meridian. It also treats constipation, headaches and the urinary system.

St 38: midway down the calf, just on the outer side of the muscle beside the shin bone below St 36. For treating shoulder pain.

St 40: about two finger-widths out (towards the edge) from 38, for calming generally – whether reducing excess chi

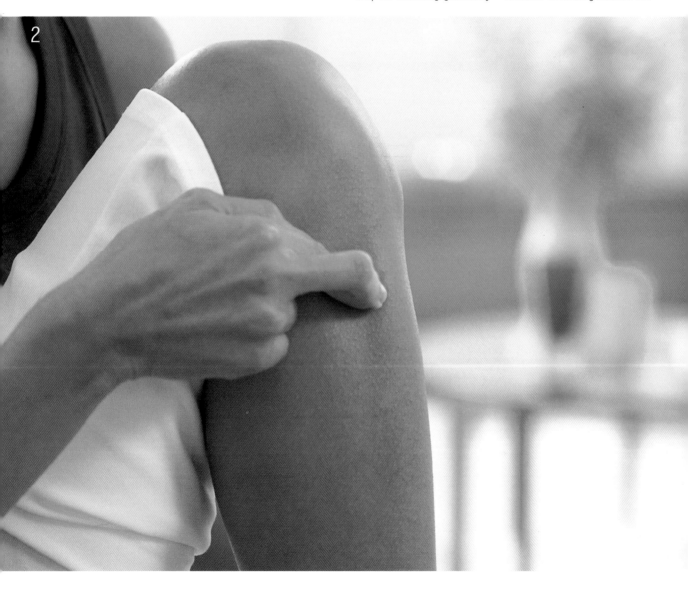

or alleviating nervous feelings. Press and hold this point for several seconds while breathing out, to calm your nerves when you are anxious and to reduce excess energy in the body.

St 41: in the ankle, for ankle pain. Flex your foot to find the crease. On the crease, this point is a natural dip half way from the ankle bone to the front of the ankle.

SPLEEN MERIDIAN

The spleen meridian runs upwards from the big toe to the armpits. It is associated with learning and concentration, and transforms the energy from food into chi.

Sp 1: the bottom inside corner of the big toenail. For treating headaches.

Sp 4: the end of the big toe bone below the bulge on the side of the foot. This is good for pain in the foot, but also benefits the reproductive system and promotes fertility.

Sp 6: four finger-widths up the inner leg from the ankle bone, starting from the fleshy area behind the ankle bone. This is a very big energy point where three meridians cross.
Warning: do not use this point during pregnancy.

Sp 9: on the inside of the calf, just under the bulge of bone below the side of the knee. For leg problems, fluid retention and varicose veins.

Sp 10: the width of two thumbs above the knee starting from the inner edge of the knee cap. Used to treat various skin conditions and also as a local point for knee pain.

Sp 12: in the crease where the front of the thigh joins the body, just beside the vulva.

Sp 13: close to Sp 12, slightly farther towards the outside of the body. Sp 12 and 13 can be used to ease period pain.

Sp 21: five fingers down from your armpit, between the fifth and sixth rib. This clears pain in the chest and helps to relieve depression.

HEART MERIDIAN

The heart meridian runs from the top of the arm to the hand. It is associated with the mind and long-term memory. It is rarely used for self-treatment, other than through meridian massage and H 7.

H 7: directly below the bony prominence of the wrist on the little finger side – the outer edge of the front of the wrist. This can be used for calming and is often used for this purpose in acupuncture.

SMALL INTESTINE MERIDIAN

The small intestine meridian runs up the arm and shoulder from the little finger to the edge of the jawbone. It is linked to the heart and is useful for clearing all kinds of blockages.

SI 3: on the outer edge of the hand just below the little finger joint. For rheumatism.

SI 9: behind the ball and socket joint of the shoulder.

SI 10: just above the inside of the armpit. Both SI 9 and SI 10 are very good for relieving shoulder pain.

BLADDER MERIDIAN

The bladder meridian runs down the back a couple of finger-widths away from the spine, and transforms fluids. Massaging the long muscles that run down the length of the spine works many bladder points.

Bl 1: in the eye socket beside the inner edge of the eye. For eye problems.

Bl 2: pinch the bridge of the nose just below the end of the eyebrow. Often used for eye problems and for calming nerves and energy.

Bl 11: find the big bone at the nape of the neck and press just below the outer edges of it. This is good for the lungs.

Bl 15: between the shoulder blades, below the fifth thoracic vertebra. For calming the heart.

Bl 23: hands on waist, thumbs on the big muscles beside the spine. Working on this point improves the circulation of blood around the body and chi to the kidneys and to the back in general.

Bl 40: behind the knee in the middle. For sciatica.

KIDNEY MERIDIAN

The kidney meridian goes up the body from the sole of the foot to the top of the chest. The body's source energy – the chi we are born with – is stored in this meridian, which also governs growth, will power and short-term memory.

Ki 1: the centre of the foot just below the ball of the foot in the middle, where the two parts meet. Called the 'bubbling spring', this important point contains a lot of energy. It is also the Earth chakra, which balances the whole body. For calming distress or dizziness.

Ki 27: under the collar bones right beside the breast bone – another calming point. Rubbing this spot helps ease coughs and asthma, so it is a good place to rub in remedies such as eucalyptus oil.

PERICARDIUM MERIDIAN

Known as the 'heart protector', the pericardium meridian runs from the chest to the middle finger. Press the end point of this meridian, under the top of the middle fingernail, to treat anxiety, tension or shock.

Pc 6: three finger-widths down the wrist, press with the third finger, right in the centre. (For many people, this is under the buckle of their watch strap.) It cures dizziness and nausea from various causes including drug side effects or following surgery.

Pc 8: the middle of the palm. It is known as the gateway of the body's energies. Healers radiate energy from this spot.

TRIPLE ENERGISER MERIDIAN

The triple energiser meridian is concerned with regulating warmth and balancing the body's fluid levels between the kidney and the heart, so stimulating the lymph system. This meridian runs from the ring finger to the eyebrow.

TE 3: halfway down the back of the hand between ring and little fingers.

TE 5: three finger-widths down from the wrist on the back of your arm (opposite Pc 6).

TE 17: in the dip behind the ear.

GALL BLADDER MERIDIAN

The gall bladder is a long meridian that runs from the head to the tip of the little toe.

GB 14: halfway up the forehead from the middle of each eyebrow. For headaches and eyestrain.

GB 20: on the base of the skull at the back, two points about four finger-widths apart, beside the top of the spine – nod your head to feel the two big muscles, then press in at the outside of them at the hairline. These points are good for headaches, colds, sinusitis and congestion in the head.

GB 30: on the side of the buttock. Put your thumbs on your hip bones, stretch your little fingers around the back and find the spot where your middle fingers ends. For hip pain.

GB 31: mid-thigh, on the outside of the leg. For sciatica.

GB 34: just below the knee. Feel for a dip between the large shinbone, the tibia, and the smaller fibula. It is just below the knobbly top of the tibia. Eases muscle pain.

LIVER MERIDIAN

The liver meridian runs from the big toes to the chest and regulates the flow of chi.

Liv 3: between the big and second toes, two finger-widths up the foot from the join between the toes. For hypertension.

GOVERNOR VESSEL

The governor vessel (also known as governor channel – a channel or vessel is a meridian) runs from just above the anus to the upper lip. Points are on the spine itself, just below the bony prominences, whereas the bladder points are beside the spine.

GV 4: at the back of the waist, between the vertebrae. For increasing vitality.

GV 14: on the big bone at the nape of the neck. Bend the head forward to find the highest point of that bone. A good energy point for pain in the upper body and rheumatism.

GV 20 (not used in this book) is on top of the head where all the meridians meet. The most yang part of the body. **Warning:** it should not be touched on anyone who has hypertension, since it may raise blood pressure.

GV 26: the end point is just below the nose, on the upper lip. Good for cases of shock or severe back pain.

CONCEPTION VESSEL

The conception vessel is a line down the centre front of the body, from the roof of the mouth.

CV 1: the beginning of this channel, a point on the perineum between the sexual organs and the anus. The most yin part of the body.

CV 4: four finger-widths below the navel. A good point for restoring vitality.

CV 6: 'sea of energy', two finger-widths below the navel. For centring and 'grounding', fertility and sexual energy.

CV 17: The heart point, or 'sea of tranquillity'. Between the breasts, three thumb-widths up from the bottom of the breastbone. This point is an important energy point and can ease heart problems.

CV 22: between the collar bones, in the salt cellar – the dip between the collarbones. Good for phlegm, sore throats and tightness in the chest.

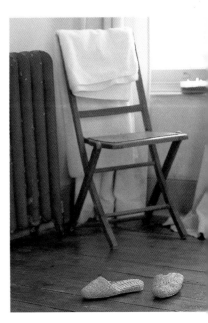

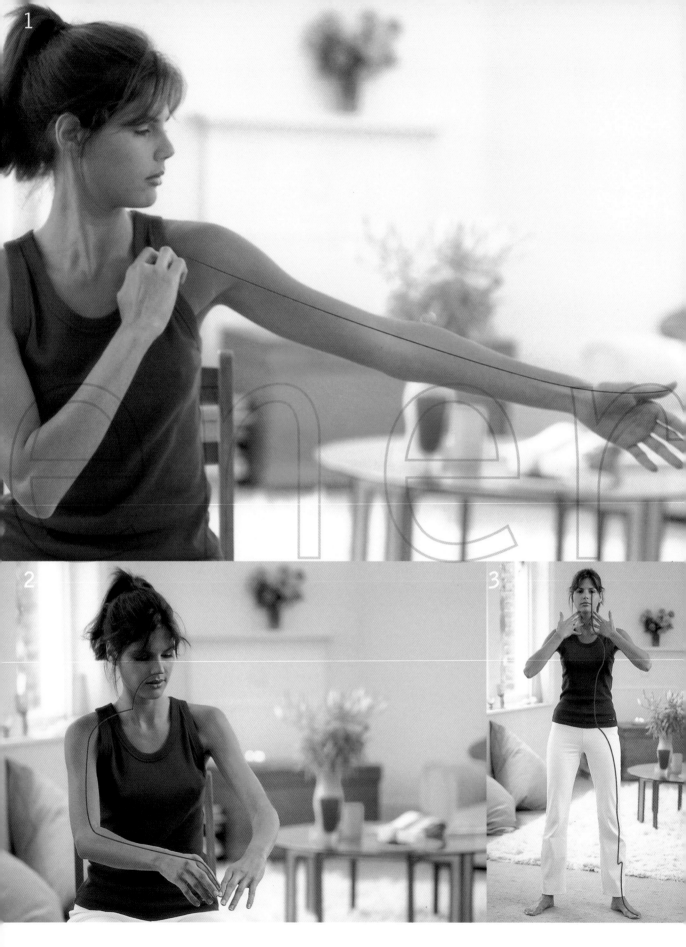

opening the energy gates

Balance all your systems with this simple daily meridian massage. It can be done in one go at any time of day. However, since the meridians and their organs are most active at certain times of the day (working on a body clock) you could also do the paired exercises as near as possible to the appropriate times – fitting in with Western advice to take work breaks.

The meridians run in different directions, but you don't necessarily have to follow their flow – you can work both up and down. Stroking is effective, while tapping or massaging give more invigorating results.

Make sure you work both sides of the body. You can go down one side and up the other, or up and down the same side and then the other side. However, it is simplest to work on both sides at the same time with mirrored movements. As you get used to the simple, flowing style you will develop a swinging rhythm that enhances the relaxing, balancing effect

Early in the morning, wake up by working on the lung meridian, which is most active between 3 and 5am, and the large intestine, between 5 and 7am. In practice, this means working these two meridians soon after you wake.
Lung: start inside the edge of the chest just below the collarbones (1). Work straight down the top of the arm (holding your hand out, looking at the palm) to the thumb.
Large intestine: from the tip of the index finger (2) up the back of the arm, over the shoulder to the outer edge of the nose on the other side of the face.

The stomach meridian is most active between 7 and 9am, and the spleen between 9 and 11am.
Stomach: start on the front of your face just below the eyes, down the front of your body (3) – not quite centrally – over your breasts, down the front of your legs to the end of the second toe.

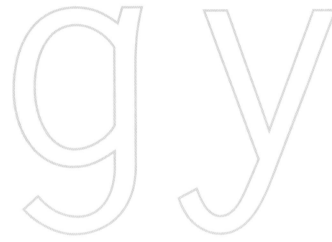

Spleen: from the tip of the big toe, up the side of the foot, up the inside of the legs, up the front of your body about a third of the way across (4), up the sides of the breasts to the armpits.

The heart meridian is most active between 11am and 1pm, and the small intestine between 1 and 3pm.
Heart: from the top of the arm just below the armpit (5) down the inside of the arm – holding your hand up as if looking at your palm – to the side of hand below the little finger. Then turn the palm down.
Small intestine: from the top of the little finger up the outside of the arm, over the shoulder as far as you can reach, up the neck, across under the ears, ending in the little hole on the edge of the face beside the jawbone (5).

The bladder meridian is most active between 3 and 5pm, and the kidney between 5 and 7pm.
Bladder: starting from the inside of the eye beside the nose, move up near the centre of the forehead, over the top of the head (6) and down beside the spine, going as far as you can reach. Below the waist, slant out slightly towards the hip and go down the back of the leg – halfway between the centre line and the outer edge – until you reach the outside of the little toe.
Kidney: starting from the sole of the foot (7) go up the inside of the legs and the front of the body a couple of finger-widths from the centre, branching out very slightly at the diaphragm, up to the top of the chest under the collarbones, close to the breast bone.

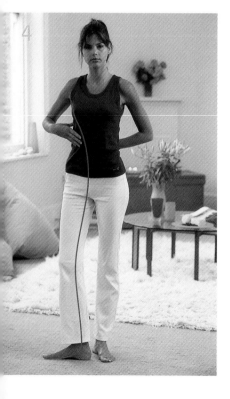

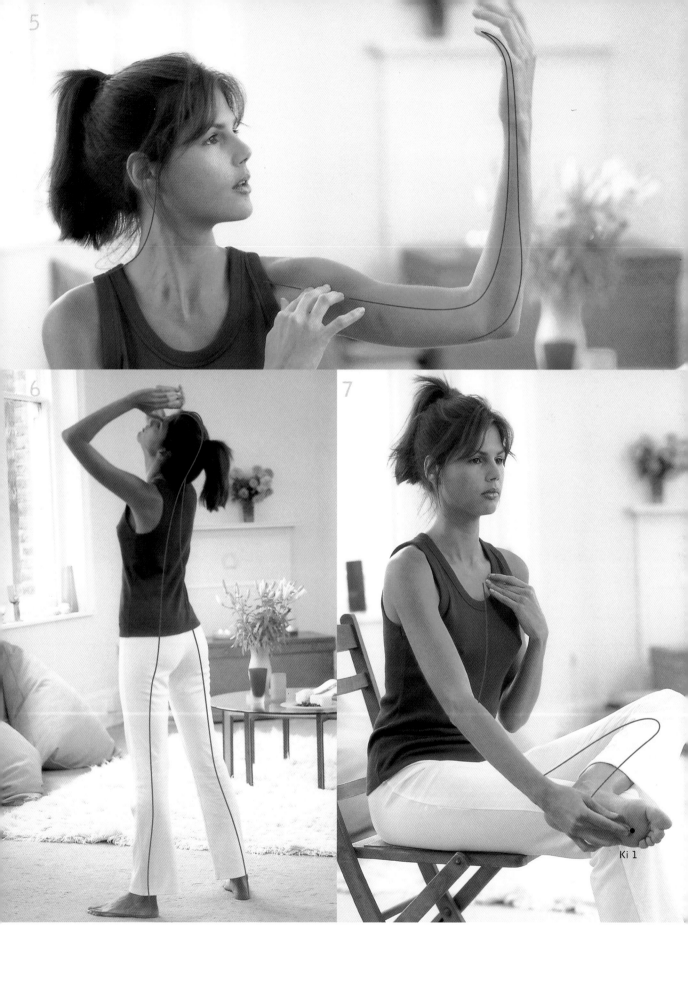

5

6

7

Ki 1

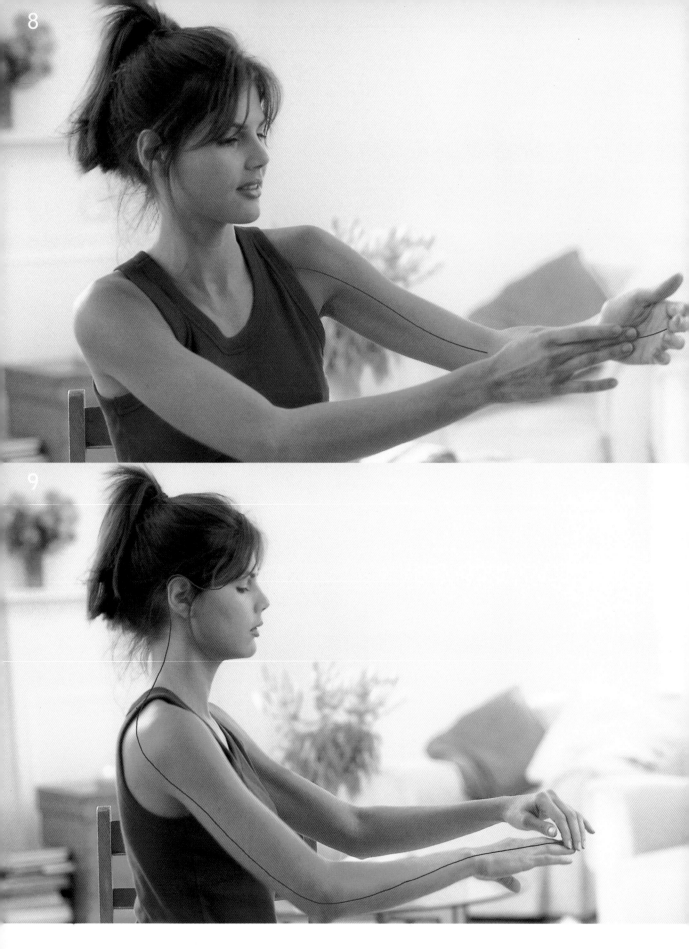

The pericardium meridian is most active between 7 and 9pm, and the triple energiser between 9 and 11pm.

Pericardium: starting from the side of the chest, down the middle of the arm (if you are holding your hand palm up) up the palm (8) to the tip of the middle finger. Turn the hand over to start the next meridian.

Triple energiser: from the tip of the ring finger (9) up the back of the hand and arm, up the side of the neck behind the ear, and over the top of the ear to the outermost tip of the eyebrow.

The gall bladder meridian is most active between 11pm and 1am, and the liver between 1 and 3am.

Gall bladder: massage the side of the head (10) and then work down the sides of the neck to the front of the chest, then work across and down the side of the body and legs to the little toe.

Liver: up from the top of the big toe, between the first and second toe bones, and the front of the legs just inside the kneecap, up to the ribs (11). Stop below the nipples.

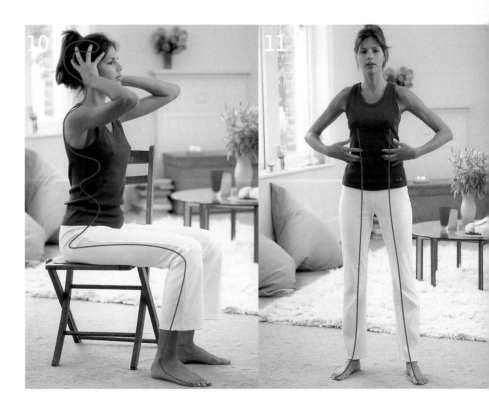

preparation

Test out the methods on yourself before trying them on anyone else: squeeze a ball; try massaging a pillow with gentle kneading motions to get a feel for the movement; practise pressing with straight fingers and tapping as if playing a piano. Relax your hands by stretching and releasing the fingers, waving them as if conducting an orchestra and shaking them from the wrist.

Remember to wash your hands both before and after carrying out a treatment, even when working on yourself. You are working with stagnation, especially where there is pain: washing your hands will help to keep your energy channels open.

techniques

Press with the flat of your palm when you are working on muscles. Massage with the pads of your fingers, not digging with fingertips (1).

Press into individual points with your index finger, or use the thumb for increased pressure. You can reinforce the pressure (2) by placing the thumb, middle and index fingers together.

Use a light touch over bony areas, which can be painful.

On the most sensitive spots, touch with the tips of your middle and index finger, without applying any pressure.

Using one finger, go in very lightly with a circular movement (3), without lifting it off the skin. Hold your

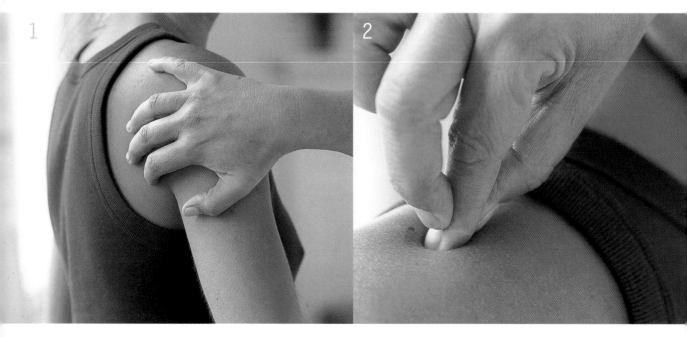

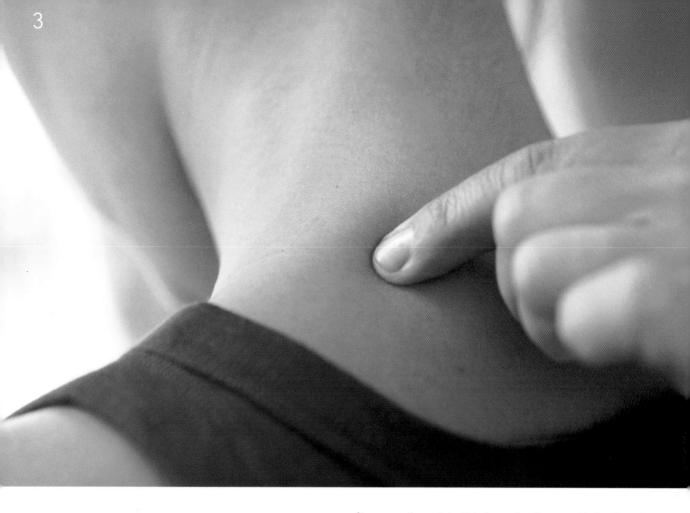

finger on the point. Reinforce the finger with the thumb and middle finger, so all three are pressing together.

Don't feel you have to dig in hard. You shouldn't cause pain, other than a brief tenderness that stops hurting when you remove the pressure. Just massaging or stroking around the area may be enough. If there is pain you can work above and below it on the same meridian, or on other meridians in the same area. If too much pain or swelling stops you going in close, you can even use the relevant meridian on the opposite side of the body.

An excellent way of working on the back meridians is to lie on a couple of soft but firm juggling balls, one on each side of the spine. Shift position to move them up and down the spine. If your spine is very stiff or you have a back condition, check with your doctor before trying this.

When you find a tender trigger point, massage gently above and below, massaging five times around it in circles with one finger before holding with gentle pressure. Continue, increasing the pressure if this does not become painful, until you are massaging in quite deeply. Then stroke down and away with a firm brushing movement to release excess energy from the area.

Reflexology and acupressure are ideal therapies for long-term problems as well as first aid, and for supporting orthodox medical treatment where necessary. For more advanced care, you may choose to have professional treatment from a qualified reflexologist or from a practitioner of acupressure or shiatsu, who may also practise acupuncture or other types of massage. However, these therapies are not intended to replace orthodox medical treatment. Many serious infections require drug treatment, while some injuries or diseases can only be successfully treated with surgery.

Only treat a condition when you are sure you know what is wrong, either because it is obvious or because it has been diagnosed by a doctor, not by any other practitioner. Always consult a doctor if you have symptoms that won't go away, even if they seem trivial.

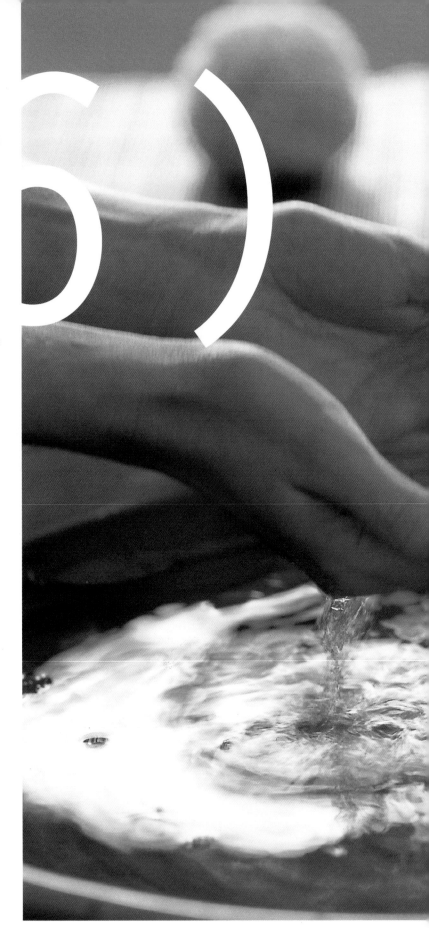

chapter six: treating problems

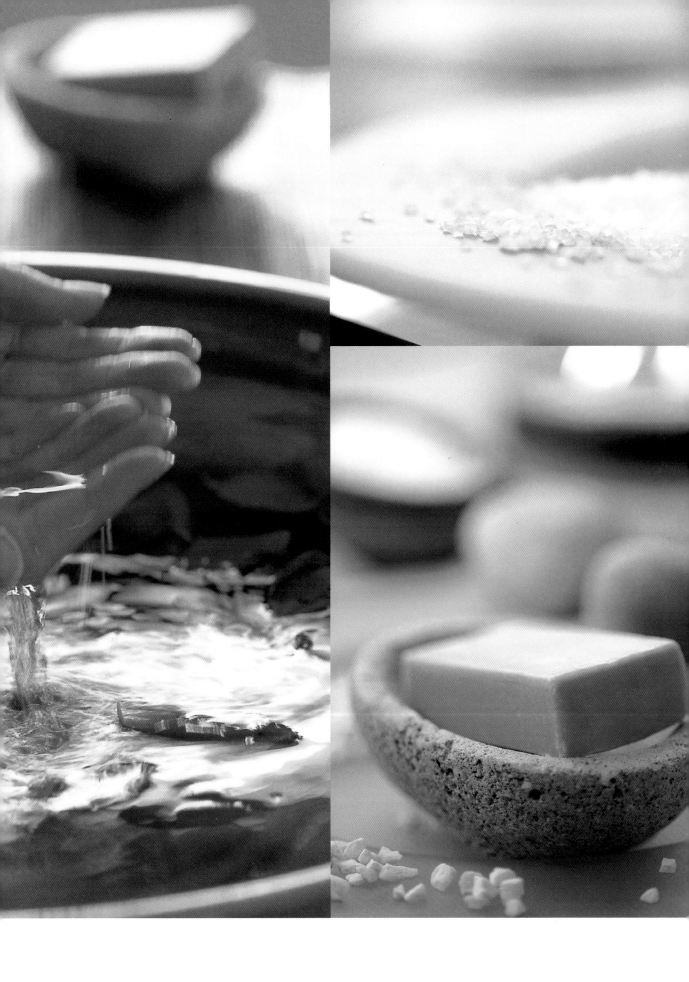

CONTRAINDICATIONS

There are problems for which even gentle techniques such as reflexology and acupressure aren't suitable, for example breast or lymphatic cancer. In these cases any massage or energy moving treatment could aid the spread of the cancer though they may be used to ease pain in terminal cancer. The first 16 weeks of pregnancy could be risky, especially in a first pregnancy or if the woman has miscarried previously. Your treatment may be harmless, but if a miscarriage occurs you will be left wondering whether it was your fault.

Don't work on cases of infectious disease, acute fever or conditions requiring surgery. Obviously you shouldn't work over a bruise, inflammation, swelling, broken skin, varicose vein or broken bone. Where the injury is on one side of the body, you can treat the appropriate point on the other side.

A fully trained and qualified reflexologist will always advise you to check with your doctor if the person being treated is taking prescription drugs, and never to overwork any individual area. A good rule is not to work any area longer than a few minutes on any one day, except in the case of first aid, when you may want to repeat the treatment briefly but frequently.

Some reflexologists advise against working with heart conditions. And don't use reflexology with any condition that damages the feet or could pass on infection; work on the hands in this case. People with diabetes often have very poor circulation, which can damage the hands and particularly the feet. Work gently without causing pain.

Acupressure isn't suitable in cases of phlebitis – inflammation of the veins often accompanied by potentially dangerous blood clots. Don't use LI 4 or Sp 6 during pregnancy, since there's a risk they might cause miscarriage, and be careful when massaging the kidney meridian not to put pressure where it crosses Sp 6. Take care when giving a head massage, since an acupressure point that can raise blood pressure is on top of the head.

If you have any serious medical conditions, check with your doctor and with a reflexology or acupressure practitioner, and only go ahead if both agree it is safe.

Remember, too, that the philosophy behind these treatments is holistic. When your shoulders ache because you don't take enough work breaks, it is of little use massaging the reflexes on your feet and assiduously working SI 9 and SI 10. These may ease the present pain, but they won't turn you into an indestructible robot or prevent you from getting repetitive strain injury. As any practitioner will advise, you need to change the things that are causing your health problems.

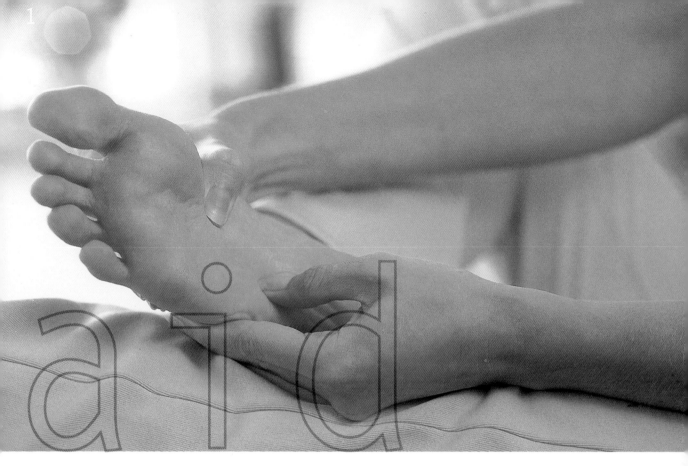

first aid

Reflexology and acupressure can be helpful when administering first aid for the following conditions. Always remember, however, that there are certain procedures that should be followed when giving first aid. The Red Cross and St John's Ambulance run courses offering certificates. If you are not a qualified first aider, then keep a first aid manual handy in the house and car at all times. Remember too to send for medical assistance in an emergency.

Once you have carried out first aid after an accident, encourage the patient to stay calm and breathe fully into the abdomen. Shocks and injuries fill the body with adrenaline that, if it can't be used to fight or run away, causes tension and increases the pain.

ASTHMA AND ALLERGIES

If you see someone having an asthma attack or serious allergic reaction, ask if they have relevant drugs with them. Stay calm, but be ready to get medical help quickly. If you are having an attack, try to use breathing exercises as for pain relief. It is a good idea to practise between attacks so you get into the habit of breathing out fully rather than trying to gasp in air.

Reflexology

During an asthma attack, work on the endocrine system, paying special attention to the adrenal (see 1) and pituitary glands. Then work on the solar plexus, diaphragm, lungs and bronchi to release the spasm in the chest, and the master gland, the pituitary, which normalises the endocrine system. If the person is producing a lot of mucus, work on the ileocaecal valve (1) to normalise mucus production.

Allergies need similar care, especially if the attack causes spasm and a streaming nose. Also, work on any other areas affected by the allergy, and on the hypothalamus. Since this is a hypersensitive reaction, do extra work on the adrenals to help normalise the response.

Acupressure

Use soothing pressure over the upper back – this can be especially helpful for children. GV 14 can help, and there's a special point for asthma on either side of the big bone at the base of the neck that stands out when you tip your head forwards.

Warning: don't try to treat asthma or any other acute respiratory attack without getting medical advice.

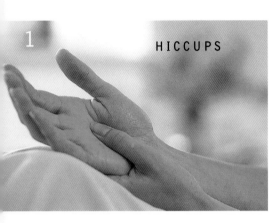

1   HICCUPS

HICCUPS

Hiccups can be irritating, but are not usually a threat to health. Both reflexology and acupressure may be helpful.

Reflexology

You may be able to stop an attack of hiccups by working first with the digestive system, then on the glottis, oesophagus, solar plexus (1), diaphragm, the chest area, lungs and heart.

Acupressure

Press into TE 17, located in the dip behind the earlobe, and hold this for a minute or so while you sit down, trying to breathe deeply. Then gently hold CV 17 and CV 22 for another minute or so.

SICKNESS

If you have eaten something that has caused the sickness, vomiting is the natural, healthy response as the body tries to get rid of it. In this case, don't try to prevent the vomiting but make sure the person affected drinks plenty of water to replenish lost fluids. Ginger is surprisingly effective against all kinds of sickness, in whatever form you prefer: crystallized ginger is especially handy when you are travelling.

Reflexology

Reflexology can help the process by bringing balance back to the digestive tract. Finger-walk down the oesophagus, gently press and rotate on the stomach area and work both ways over the intestines. Finish by working the colon and rectum. If the vomiting has been severe and accompanied by cramps, do additional work – including the spinal nerves that feed the stomach and abdominal areas – and include work on the diaphragm too. Make sure you use plenty of soothing massage strokes between working on the specific areas.

To treat travel sickness, start by working the whole digestive system (1) as above, using hand reflexology if you are doing this for yourself so that you don't have to cramp your stomach while working your foot. Return to the solar plexus and pituitary gland points, rotating your thumb on them. Thumb-walk across the diaphragm and the middle and upper spine. If vertigo is involved, make several passes along the whole spine from brain to coccyx. To treat the stomach area in particular, walk down the centre of the right foot, covering the main reflex areas for the duodenum and the pylorus. This is usually carried out more easily on the hands.

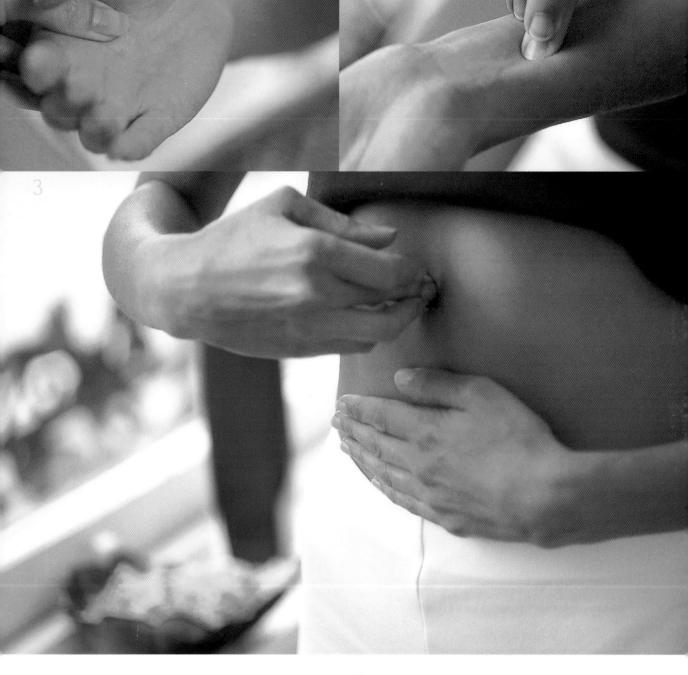

Acupressure

Pc 6 (2) is the most reliable energy remedy for all kinds of sickness, proven to be so effective that it is even being used in hospitals. For travel sickness, you can buy wrist straps that work on this point. Otherwise, just hold the point three finger-widths down the middle of the inner arm from the wrist. CV 12 (3) is another point which is very effective in easing feelings of nausea.

1

INJURIES

2

1

SHOCK

INJURIES

First aid is most important for minor injuries: ice to cool a burn, a pad pressed on the spot to stop bleeding, or RICE (rest, ice, compression, elevation) for sprains and sports' injuries. Don't move anyone if you are not sure how badly injured they are, especially if it is an older person who has fallen down.

When everything is under control, some reflexology or acupressure techniques can soothe the sufferer and help the body start the healing process.

Warning: don't use self-help techniques on anyone who has, or may have, serious injuries such as a broken bone or internal bleeding. Just send for an ambulance, help the injured person to remain calm and don't try to move them. If they are unconscious, keep checking that they are breathing.

Reflexology

Start by working the endocrine system, then concentrate on the solar plexus and diaphragm to counteract the stress caused by an injury.

For a nose bleed (1), press firmly between the nail and joint of the big toe – the nose reflex – while the person sits with their head forwards and pinches the bridge of their nose. Work their whole foot from toes to heels to help bring energy down the body and reduce pressure in the head. For self-help, you can carry out the same procedure on the hand that is pinching your nose.

Acupressure

Touch lightly on the nearest meridian above or below any injuries (2, for example for shoulder pain) and hold for as long as is comfortable.

SHOCK

If someone seems shaken after a mishap, check to see that they are not hurt more seriously than was originally thought. If they appear confused, even after an apparently minor accident, get medical help immediately. Keep them warm; you can give them water or sweet tea to drink if you are absolutely certain that they do not have a physical injury. Otherwise do not offer any food or drink.

Use the remedies below while you are waiting for medical help to arrive: work gently and soothingly, making sure you are not hurting any injured part.

Reflexology

Work on the endocrine system, paying particular attention to the adrenal reflexes. Help to 'earth' the sufferer by working down the spine reflexes from the big toe and stroking the whole foot from the toes to the ankles, encouraging the movement of energy back into the whole body. Sometimes holding the heel firmly with one hand while keeping your other thumb over the pituitary point (1) helps to even out the flow of energy in the spine. Encourage this by visualising energy or white light flowing down the spine. Don't forget that you can work on the hands too, which may be more soothing in these circumstances.

The same routine can help someone who is feeling faint or sick or is vomiting.

Acupressure

Any of the calming points can be used to soothe the patient suffering from shock caused by accidents. St 40 (2) is particularly effective. Press and hold for several seconds while breathing out as slowly as possible. Press under the fingernails or toenails with your own nail, especially the middle fingernail where the pericardium meridian ends; this can also help if the shock has made the patient lose their voice. Ki 1 (a grounding point that connects you to the Earth) and GV 26 are particularly helpful for shock. Ki 1 is excellent for dizziness too: just putting your feet flat on the floor can help, or get someone to put their middle fingers on the spot just below the centre of the ball of your foot.

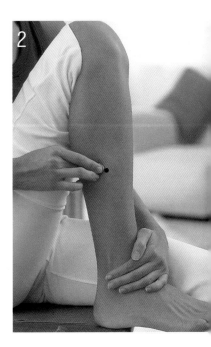

soothing pain

Pain relief was the earliest use of modern reflexology, when, before the body's zones had been identified, Dr Fitzgerald found he could produce numbness by applying pressure to the ears or lips. A reflexologist's tiny movements encourage release of tension in distant parts of the body in the same zone.

Reflexologists and acupressurists try to find the cause of the pain and treat that, since the aim of holistic therapies is to solve the root problem rather than just easing symptoms. For example, constant headaches can as easily be caused by digestive problems, anxiety, insomnia, an undiagnosed illness or bad posture – and each of these in turn can be caused by a number of factors, all of which need to be addressed.

Many of us accept pain – from conditions such as arthritis – as an inevitable part of growing older, choosing to treat the symptoms rather than seeking a cure for the condition that causes the pain. However, it is far better to

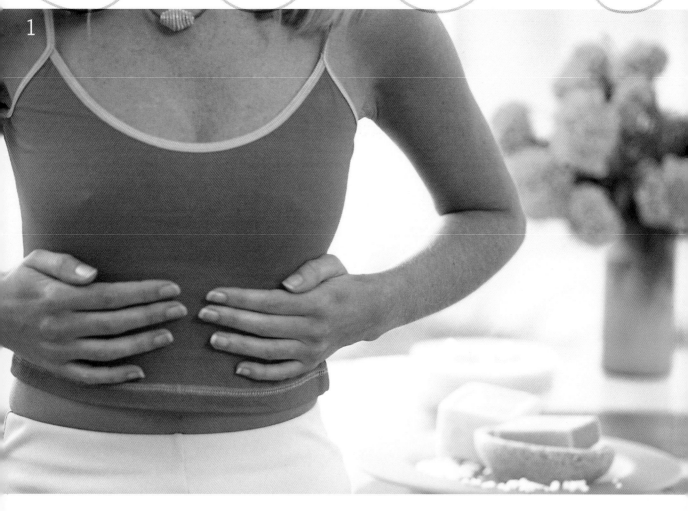

1

visit the GP to see if something can be done. And where orthodox medicine cannot help, complementary therapies may. Arthritis, for example, often responds to food supplements such as glucosamine sulphate, digestive problems to dietary changes and back pain to a good, qualified chiropractor.

At the same time, use full reflexology and acupressure treatments to try to get at the root cause, as well as the specific pain-relieving moves given in this section.

Relaxation techniques are important for pain reduction: any kind of pain causes us to tense our muscles, even though this may make us feel worse, so include the treatments given in this book for stress. It is difficult to relax when something is hurting, yet this is the best way to ease the pain, going with it rather than uselessly confronting it and increasing tension. It not only eases the element of pain that has been caused physically by tension, but reduces the pain's powerful psychological hold. Simply sitting quietly and visualising tension flowing like water out of your whole body is a good start.

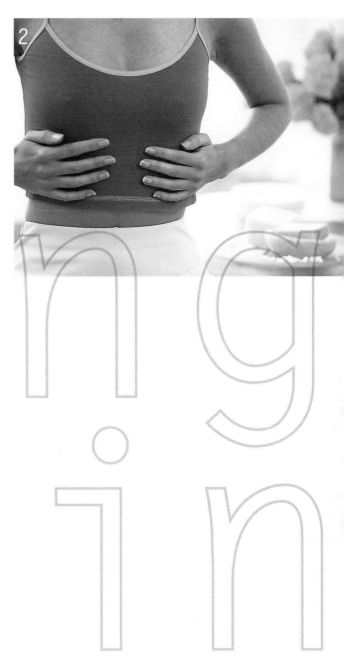

BREATHING

Breathing exercises also help to control the pain. Just learning to breathe slowly and letting the breath out fully can help reduce levels of adrenaline (the fight-or-flight hormone, produced during physical or psychological stress) that makes pain feel worse. Let your breath slow down naturally. Then put your hands side by side on your abdomen, fingertips meeting below the navel (1). Breathe in through your nose, to the count of four, and feel the oxygen pushing your hands apart (2).

Breathe out through your mouth to the count of at least six, ensuring the lungs are empty. If you are alone, make a long sighing noise as you let the breath out. If it is comfortable to do so, let your lungs stay empty for a few seconds before breathing in again.

Warning: check with your doctor before doing any breathing exercise if you have epilepsy or high blood pressure, and stop if you start feeling light-headed – you have been breathing too deeply.

Any pain of unknown origin should be investigated. Even if it wears off, it could still mean you have a condition that requires medical attention.

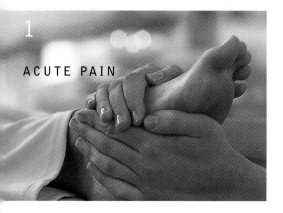

ACUTE PAIN

ACUTE PAIN

The mind is as powerful as the body when it comes to dealing with pain. Waxing your legs can hurt like anything, but somehow the pain is nowhere near as painful as, for example, having the dressing changed on a nasty wound. In the same way, a dentist's injection is much worse than having your ears pierced. The things we do for beauty may actually create a stronger physical sensation, but the circumstances aren't distressing, so any momentary pain doesn't trouble us. Since our natural feelings of panic and dismay when we are gripped by sudden pain make it harder to bear, it is vital to let these go. Breathing exercises are a big help here.

Acute pain is usually caused by some kind of accident, so the first thing to do is make the person safe and give first aid. If the cause of the pain is unknown, you'll need to get medical help. Encourage the sufferer to stay calm and breathe fully into the abdomen. Shocks and accidents fill the body with stress hormones which, if they can't be used to fight or run away, cause tension and increase the pain.

Reflexology

A soothing massage (1) will start helping to ease the pain before you even reach any specific points. Pain causes spasm, so help the body relax by working on the solar plexus and diaphragm points – simultaneously encouraging the patient to take some long, slow breaths with you. Next work the endocrine system, paying particular attention to the pituitary point to normalise glandular activity. Massaging the point in the big toe that represents the hypothalamus will normalise the response of the sympathetic nervous system, especially if you also work along the spine from top to bottom – from toe to heel – to calm the nerves carrying the pain message. Work on the adrenals will encourage the production of soothing hydrocortisone, which will also calm any inflammation or allergic reaction.

Next, work on the specific points for the area that hurts, to normalise circulation.

Acupressure

Press and hold LI 4. Also work on trigger points: find the spot that hurts and gently rub above and below at first, to unblock stagnant energy. Then move onto the spot and rub in small circles three or four times – but not hard enough to cause more pain – then continue the movement by stroking down and away from the pain. Repeat several times. This is a very gentle and soothing way to ease a child's pain.

CHRONIC PAIN

When pain becomes part of our lives we often build up patterns of tension that become hard to break, especially if we have no idea that we are doing it. Gentle massage by a friend or family member can go a long way towards reducing the debilitating, exhausting effects of chronic pain. Many people who would not consider a full body massage enjoy the relaxing effects of massage on their hands, feet or head and shoulders. Breathing exercises can also be helpful.

Reflexology

When carrying out reflexology, work over the whole foot so that the small movements encourage tissue to release the built-up tension. Thumb- and finger-walk the bony ridges along the length of the side of the foot to release tension in the spine and back muscles. Work across the top of the foot, paying extra, gentle, attention to any parts that are sensitive. The diaphragm is important, as it restores normal breathing – we tend to breathe shallowly when we are in pain. Working on the solar plexus and diaphragm (1) helps relax and move excess energy away from the painful area.

Specific moves, after the main treatment, include the solar plexus and diaphragm points to relieve spasm, the hypothalamus to calm the pain-bearing nerves and the adrenals to ease any inflammation. Work on the reflexes for the painful area and the spine from toes to heels.

Acupressure

Hold the hand over the centre of the pain to calm it, then stroke away from it to encourage excess energy away from the spot. Encourage the person to keep breathing the pain out as you work.

Use LI 4, the 'great eliminator', for all pain in the upper body (see page 66). Sp 21 (2) is good for boosting the immune system against the debilitating effects of chronic pain. Put your thumb in your armpit, spread your hand down the side of your chest and press the point on your side where your middle finger ends.

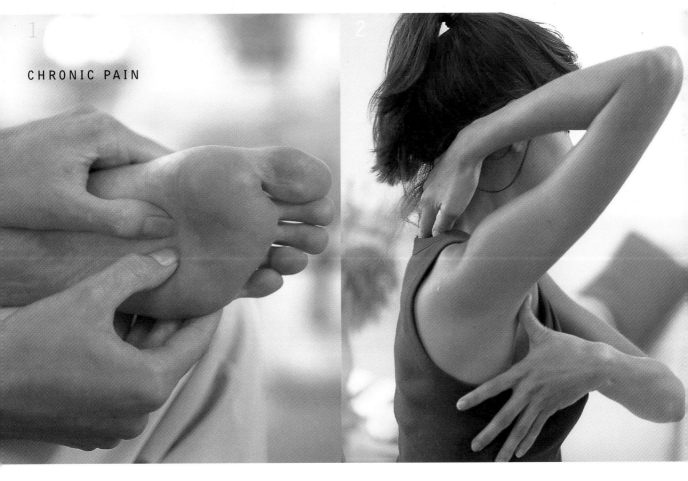

CHRONIC PAIN

HEADACHES

When the work you are doing causes a headache, go for a walk and get some fresh air – if headaches are frequent, try to do this in time to defuse them. Check your posture; if your shoulders are hunched or if you are straining your eyes, headaches will be inevitable.

Try to visualise breathing out pain as you carry out these treatments. Cup your palms over your eyes for a minute or so to rest them after doing any work around them (1).

Reflexology

Thumb- or finger-walk all over the pad of the big toe – this is also said to stimulate the brain. If a headache is caused by sinuses, squeeze the sides and back of each toe (2). A tired headache across the forehead can be eased by pressing just below the big toenail (3).

Acupressure

Different parts of the head relate to different meridians and blockages. All the meridians pass through the neck, so a neck massage often eases the problem wherever it started. Concentrate on the hairline at the base of the skull. Also work on the trigger points, gently moving the skin in circles, then stroking the energy down and away. Find the 'third eye' point, in the centre of the forehead between the eyebrows or just above that point. Feel for a natural, tiny dip.

You can also ease headaches by working on the hands or feet. For hands, start from the wrist below your little finger and run the opposite index finger up and down the sides of the fingers as if drawing an outline of your hand, ending at the bottom of the thumb. Pull each finger and thumb as if pulling a cap off it. Work your way around all the fingernails by pressing in with your fingernail. This opens the meridians. Massaging the foot can encourage excess energy away from the head, relieving local pain.

If there is eyestrain as well, rub up and down between points Bl 1 and Bl 2 from the inner corner of the eye nearly up to the eyebrow, and GB 14 above the centre of each eyebrow, halfway to your hairline. Tap or massage around the bone under the eyebrow.

MIGRAINE

Try to work out what brings on a migraine so you can avoid it or, if unavoidable, take steps in advance to mitigate it. Properly supervised exclusion diets sometimes work when all else fails. Prevention is better than cure, so seek qualified treatment from a specialist such as an acupuncturist or physiotherapist. Migraine often has other symptoms, so you may also need to work on points for eye strain, dizziness or nausea.

Reflexology

Massage the brain and central nervous system in the big toe, then concentrate on the head, neck and shoulder reflexes. The neck muscles (1) are on one side of the big toe, next to the second toe; the vertebrae (2) are on the other side, where they continue the spine down the inner edge of the foot.

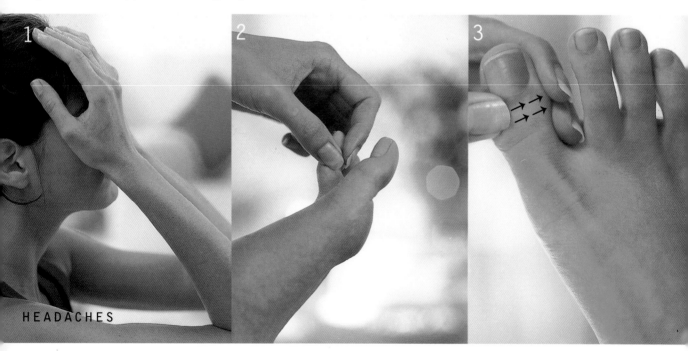

HEADACHES

MIGRAINE

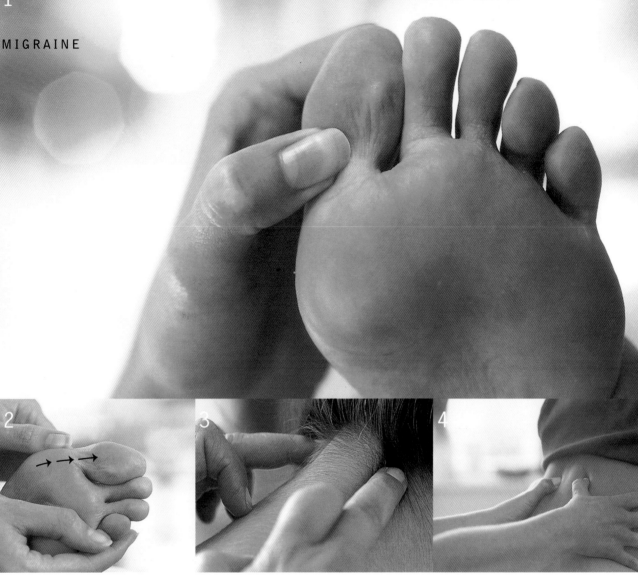

Migraine is often triggered by food, so work on the digestive system to start with. Then move to the head area, including the hypothalamus and pituitary gland, and the spine – often the seat of tension that leads to headaches.

Acupressure

Find pain points halfway down the top of the hand, between the second and third, and the fourth and fifth hand bones. Use light pressure, pulling the fingers away from the head. Work the back of the neck, GB 20 (3) at the base of the skull: nod your head a few times to feel where this is and find a point on the outside of the muscle beside the spine.

Massage the back beside the spine and above the waist, pushing gently outwards and downwards, to work on bladder point BL 20 (4). Also work on St 40, Sp 6, Pc 6 and GB 14, halfway up the forehead from the middle of each eyebrow. Circle and press five times.

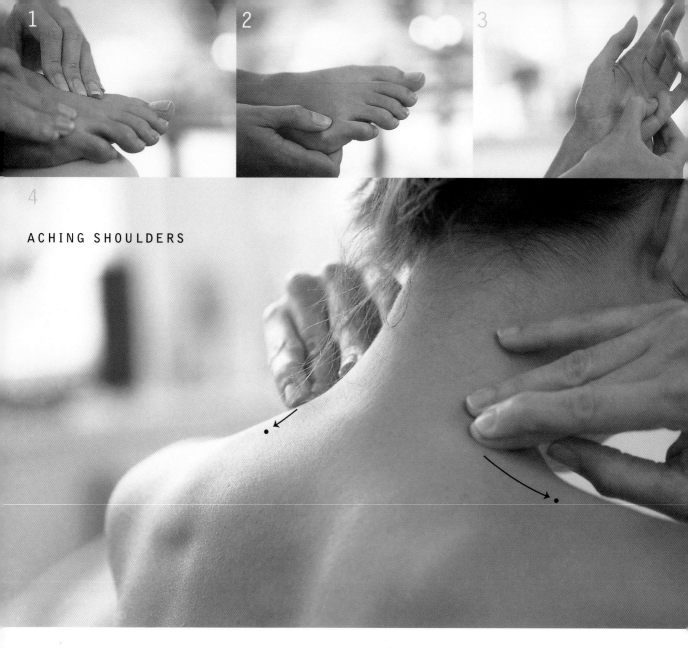

ACHING SHOULDERS

ACHING SHOULDERS

Aching shoulders are almost always caused by strain, and can in most cases be relieved by improving your posture. Try Alexander Technique or Feldenkrais classes.

Reflexology

Knead (1) and massage your way across both the top and the sole of the foot, about 25mm (1 in) from the toes. Pinch, press and gently hold for a count of five on the shoulder point located on the foot (2) between the bases of the fourth and fifth toes and on the hand between the bases of the fourth and fifth fingers (3).

Acupressure

To ease stiff shoulders, press gently GB 21 (4) on top of the shoulder, in the middle of the slope between the shoulder and neck, while the person you are working on breathes out and visualises pain leaving the spot. LI 11, LI 4, St 38, SI 9 and SI 10 can also help.

BACK ACHE

Like aching shoulders, this can frequently be eased by improving your posture. High heels, a saggy mattress and furniture at the wrong height all add to the strain on our backs. But if back pain is persistent and has no obvious cause, see your GP. If the doctor rules out any medical condition, a physiotherapist, osteopath or chiropractor can often provide help.

Reflexology

On your hand, the spine runs down the edge of the thumb to just above the wrist. To work the spine, finger- or thumb-walk all the way down the bony ridge (1). To ease tired back muscles, use your four fingers and knead or walk horizontally across the bony ridge (2), searching for any sensitive areas. Finish with soothing massage strokes down the hand, covering the spinal reflexes. On your foot, the spine runs all the way down the edge of the foot.

Acupressure

Work on trigger points (where it hurts), plus GB 30 and 31. Use Bl 40 behind the knee for sciatica. Massage the bladder and gall bladder meridians – if you are working on yourself, lie on juggling balls (see page 77).

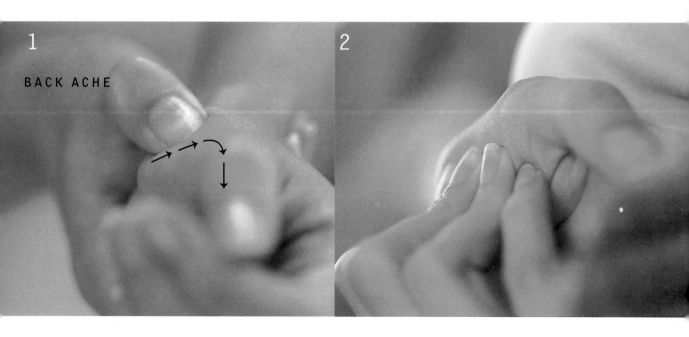

1

2

BACK ACHE

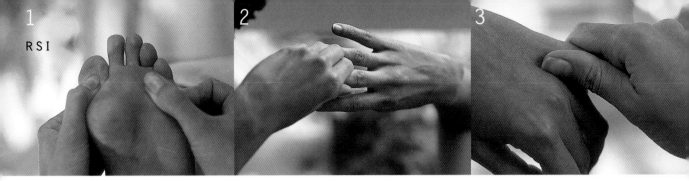

REPETITIVE STRAIN INJURY (RSI)

RSI is mainly caused by work involving constantly repeated small movements. However, few people get RSI from knitting for hours, suggesting that tension plays a part too. No workplace will ever be as relaxing as a comfy armchair at home, but stressful conditions (including harsh lighting, noise, bad management and unnecessary pressure) certainly increase the tension in our bodies. Correct work furniture helps keep the back and hands in the right position, as relaxed as possible. A variety of movement is even more important: while you are working, flex your fingers, stretch your arms out and do exaggerated backwards shoulder rolls. Take regular breaks to stretch, walk around and shake tension out of your arms. Stretch your fingers. Press your palms together like an Indian dancer, elbows out to the sides.

Reflexology

Upper limb disorders may be centred on the hands, the arms or the shoulders, but all should benefit from gentle stretching. Hand reflexology is especially helpful here, but whether you are using the hands or the feet, start by treating the musculo-skeletal and nervous systems. Then concentrate on the neck, shoulder girdle (1), arm and hand reflexes. Finally work on the hip and leg reflexes, to encourage the movement of energy down the body. When treating for RSI, make sure you interrupt the stress-holding patterns by doing extra work on the finger and toe joints, rotating and stretching them gently (2).

Acupressure

The hand treatment for headaches works well with the various forms of RSI too. Run an index finger up and down the sides of the fingers, pull each finger (3) and thumb, then lightly press your nail around all the fingernails. With the palm facing upwards, tap firmly 12 times up the forearm, then tap the inside of the elbow 12 times. Turn the arm over and tap the other side of the elbow too. Gently massage across the fold at the inside of the elbow, from the heart point at the spot where the fold ends when your arm is bent, across to the centre. These are points for releasing the energy stagnation that occurs with RSI.

TOOTHACHE

Oil of cloves or whisky on the aching tooth can numb the pain until you get to a dentist.

Reflexology

Ease toothache by thumb-walking or pressing and rotating along the jawline points, on the first joint of the big toe. More conveniently, work on the hands, starting with the finger-and-thumb walking massage routine, then thumb walking or pressing and rotating along the first joint of the thumb (1).

Acupressure

Try LI 4 and St 4 (2). There are several points on the hands that are beneficial for toothache, so a hand massage can also be helpful.

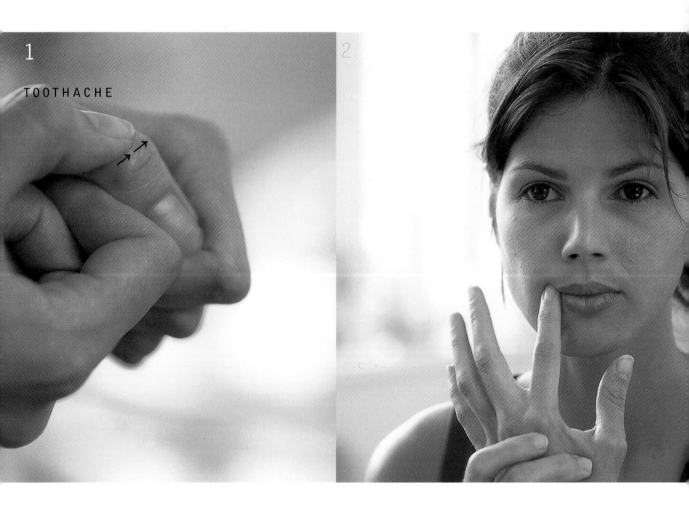

1

TOOTHACHE

2

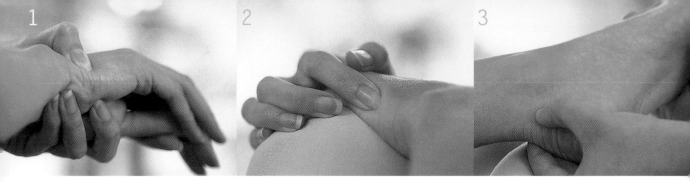

ARTHRITIS AND RHEUMATISM

These painful conditions overshadow many older people's lives, so a reflexology or acupressure treatment can be a loving gift to an elderly friend or relative. Make sure they're comfortable and relaxed before you get to work – long, gentle massage strokes are a good way to start.

Reflexology

Start by following the routine for pain, then work on the whole musculo-skeletal system and the big toe for the central nervous system. Pay special attention to the hip point (1), knees (2) or other areas that hurt, but don't risk aggravating the pain by lingering too long on them – you just want to help the energy flow. Work on the thyroid, parathyroid, adrenal and pituitary glands, and on the stomach, intestine and kidneys.

Hands and feet may both be arthritic, so work on whichever is least painful. When treating an arthritic hand or foot you will need to work very gently, avoiding all twisting and rotating movements, since these could cause damage. Thumb- and finger-walking should feel comfortable, with light pressure that may be increased as long as it doesn't cause pain.

For back pain caused by arthritis in the spine, do a chronic pain treatment, then concentrate on the spine. Massage down the side of the foot, and finger-walk across between the vertebrae points to release any nerves that may be trapped and to ease the muscle spasm that often accompanies arthritis.

Sciatica has a point of its own: draw an imaginary diagonal line from the ankle bone to the point of the heel and travel about three-quarters of the way down it, stopping where the heel bone starts. There's a sciatic reflex on each side of the heel, sitting on top of the heel bone towards the back of the foot, so hold them between finger and thumb (3). Be careful when working here, since the sciatic nerve passes over this bone and loops under the heel. If you suffer from sciatica, do this after treating the central nervous system and the spine, and then work on the hip and knee reflexes, since the nerve runs down through those joints.

Acupressure

For rheumatism, work on GV 14 and SI 3. Massage around the outside of painful joints. For back pain, massage the bladder points beside the spine, easing muscle tension too. LI 11, on the elbow, is a strong point for arthritic pain in the shoulder and arm.

For knee pain, spread the hand with the middle finger on the middle of the outer edge of the kneecap, working on St 34 above the knee, St 36 outside the knee and Sp 9 and 10 on the inner side (4). Rubbing this area also stimulates the right points – St 34, 35 and 36. Massage around the outside of the joint. Do the same around all painful joints.

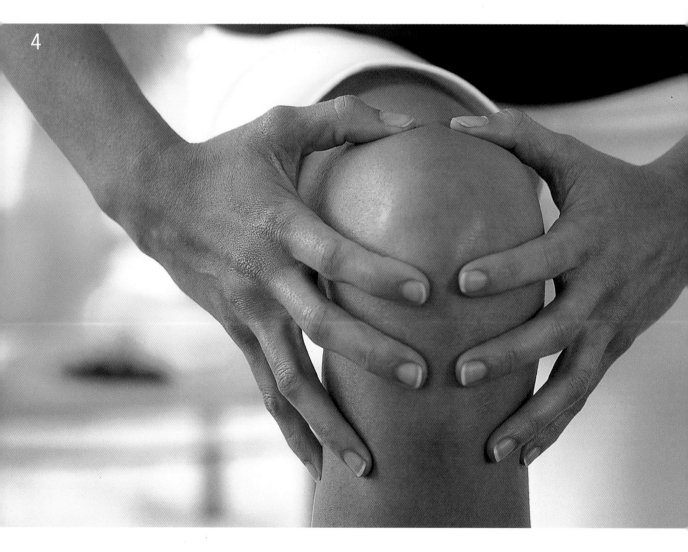

4

conditions

Self-help can improve general health and resistance to disease as well as alleviating unpleasant symptoms. It also combats the feeling of helplessness that may accompany ill-health, especially a long-term condition.

DIGESTIVE DISORDERS

If you frequently suffer from indigestion, it is a good idea not to eat fatty fast foods, drink with meals or eat a heavy meal late at night. The Hay Diet, or food combining – eating high-protein and high-carbohydrate foods at separate meals – has worked wonders for many people with digestive problems. Peppermint tea after a meal is a painless way to prevent indigestion. And don't forget stomach upsets are often caused by worry or anxiety, so try cutting down on the stress.

Reflexology

The same type of treatment works for indigestion as for sickness (see page 82). In addition, work the liver with a hook and back-up technique and pinch through on the gall

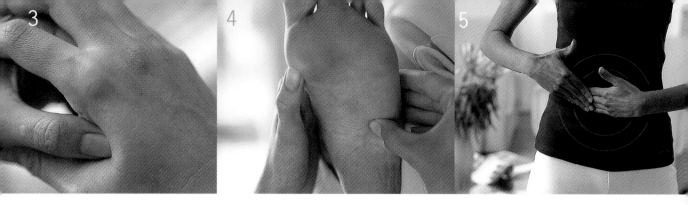

bladder reflex. Don't forget to include walking up and down the oesophagus. Include the jaw and mouth area too, since indigestion is often connected with poor salivation.

For digestive problems in general, work with the whole digestive tract starting from the mouth and following right through to the rectum. Points to concentrate on include the liver (1) and gall bladder. If you suffer cramping pains, for example with irritable bowel syndrome, work on the thyroid (2) and parathyroid (3) reflexes too, plus the diaphragm and the solar plexus.

If you suffer from food allergies, include the adrenals. For problems with sugar balance, such as hypoglycaemia or diabetes, work on the pancreas (4). To ease constipation and haemorrhoids, work on the colon, also on the area along the back of the ankle and the heel on the Achilles' tendon, known as the 'chronic helper'.

With diabetes, take care not to overwork the pancreas and check to see if medication needs adjusting, since reflexology may encourage the pancreas to produce more insulin. Some reflexologists warn that overworking the pancreas reflex could cause an insulin coma.

Acupressure

The spleen and stomach may have been affected by something harmful from outside, such as chemical additives or very spicy food.

For heartburn, work on CV 12 and LI 4. Indigestion and constipation are both eased by working on St 36 and LI 4, the great eliminator. Stomach massage also helps: clockwise from CV 6 in small circular movements for constipation (5) and anticlockwise to slow down the flow for diarrhoea. (Do this with small circular finger movements on the spot, lifting the fingers to start the next movement, working around in a big circle covering your whole abdomen from just above the navel.)

Early in the morning is the best time to massage your abdomen, as the stomach meridian is most active between 7 and 9am. However if you suffer from constipation, stomach massage can also help while you are using the lavatory; it is also worth massaging the stomach before you go to bed, so that the effects take place overnight.

1

2

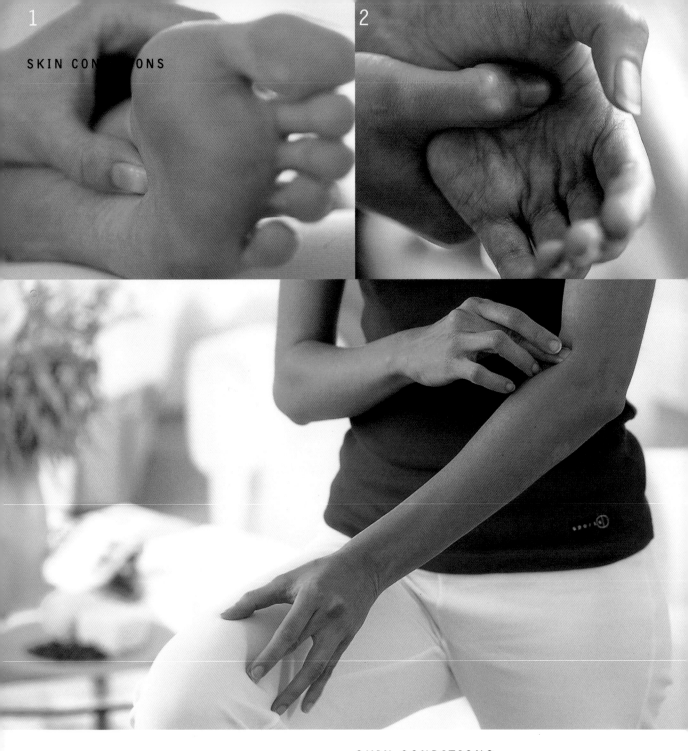

SKIN CONDITIONS

Skin is an organ of elimination as well as protection – sweat is one process by which your body gets rid of unwanted toxins. Drinking plenty of water helps keep it clear. Saturated fats may disrupt your hormonal balance, so cut down on red meat and processed foods if you are getting spotty. Eating oily fish such as mackerel and making sure you have plenty of fresh fruit and vegetables can provide the nutrients needed to keep skin healthy. Marmite is a good source of skin-friendly B vitamins.

Reflexology

If you have skin problems, work on the urinary and digestive systems first to help the process of elimination through those channels. Then pay some extra attention to the liver, bowel (1) and kidneys (2). Since some skin conditions are triggered by hormonal changes, work on the endocrine system too. In some people they are linked with overproduction of mucus, so working on the ileocaecal valve may help. Work on the face, too, by pressing below the big toenail.

Acupressure

Skin conditions are often linked with hormonal, digestive or even emotional problems that may need to be treated first. Otherwise, or in conjunction with these, try Sp 10 and LI 4 to improve your circulation, and LI 11 to aid elimination (3). The abdominal massage that aids digestion often helps clear the skin too.

CHRONIC FATIGUE SYNDROME (CFS)

CFS is more than just tiredness. (It is often called myalgic encephalomyelitis, or ME.) The constant exhaustion is just one of a range of symptoms that may include mental confusion, sweaty feet and painful sensitivity to light. One theory is that the immune system is damaged, allowing free rein to a string of infections, since it frequently follows a viral infection or a long period of overwork. Another is that the immune system is overstimulated and attacking the body. Yet another theory links the condition with chronic yeast infections. In reality, it probably has a number of different causes.

Balancing therapies such as reflexology or acupressure can do a lot for conditions such as this, for which orthodox medicine has not yet found an answer. Have a full reflexology treatment or massage all the meridians, since your aim is to work on the whole system. If you can find out what caused the illness, or is causing relapses, you can try to treat these as well. Working on the gall bladder meridian, for example, helps the body deal with pollution.

Reflexology

For best results with CFS, give 10 minutes' reflexology on each hand and foot on the same side of the body, then switch sides and treat the other hand and foot. If there isn't time to do all the systems, use the techniques for tiredness and any other symptoms.

To strengthen the immune system, work on the endocrine, lymphatic, central nervous systems and the eliminatory system, placing special emphasis on the liver and the spleen (1).

Acupressure

The previous revitalising techniques can help on a day-to-day level, as can the specific techniques for other symptoms. The 'third eye' point or 'decorating hall' (between the eyebrows) and CV 6 below the navel – the 'sea of energy' – can help ease the exhaustion, dizziness and confusion.

Massaging your back at waist level from beside the spine towards the sides (as you instinctively do if you have back ache) works on points including Bl 23 for similar effects. Pc 6 can ease nausea and heart palpitations. Two good points to help with weakness and muscle pain are just below the knee, GB 34 and St 36 – rub all around that area if you are not sure of finding the right spots.

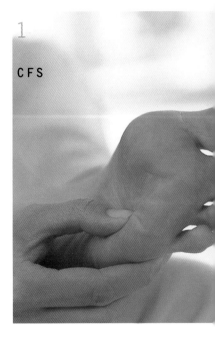

1

CFS

EXHAUSTION

Tiredness is a natural result of a long day's work, but if you are feeling constantly worn out you need to investigate the cause. If you are just tired and run down, try to reduce your workload, eat healthily and take time for some form of enjoyable relaxation. If overworking has become part of your life, you need to take a step back and reorganise your priorities. Of course that is easier said than done – but you won't be much good to anyone if you work yourself to death.

'Tired all the time' syndrome is an odd state in which you feel lethargic in spite of not having done very much. This syndrome can be caused by depression, thyroid malfunction or a number of other medical conditions, so see your GP if you suffer from this. The condition can also creep up on you if you are bored or unhappy, and perhaps feel stalled or trapped. Again, the treatments suggested here can only ease the symptoms of a problem or problems that you need to confront.

Reflexology

To help get energy moving around the body, work alternately on the hands and the feet in the same session. You may find there is very little reflex action in a very tired person. The muscle tissue may feel slack, the hands and feet may be cold and there may be a general feeling of emptiness or energy depletion in parts of the foot. There may also be little response unless the person is tense as well as tired, in which case there may well be an extra sensitivity.

If you are doing this for someone else, it is worth taking the time to do a full session, since the whole system may need to be toned up. Spend a little extra time working on any sensitive areas.

For a quicker rejuvenation, work on the endocrine system, then the adrenals (which may be exhausted), the liver, thymus (1) and the pituitary. Moving away from the feet, try tapping the breastbone, just below the collar bones, to stimulate the thymus gland (2).

Acupressure

Work Ki 1 on the sole of the foot, the 'bubbling spring'. St 36 is a great energy point just below the knee and Sp 21 is also useful. To restore some vitality and a sense of balance when you are feeling drained, sit with your feet placed flat on the floor, pressing one palm on the small of your back to cover GV 4, and the other palm below your navel to cover CV 4. Imagine that you are breathing out fatigue, breathing in a golden light that spreads energy throughout your body.

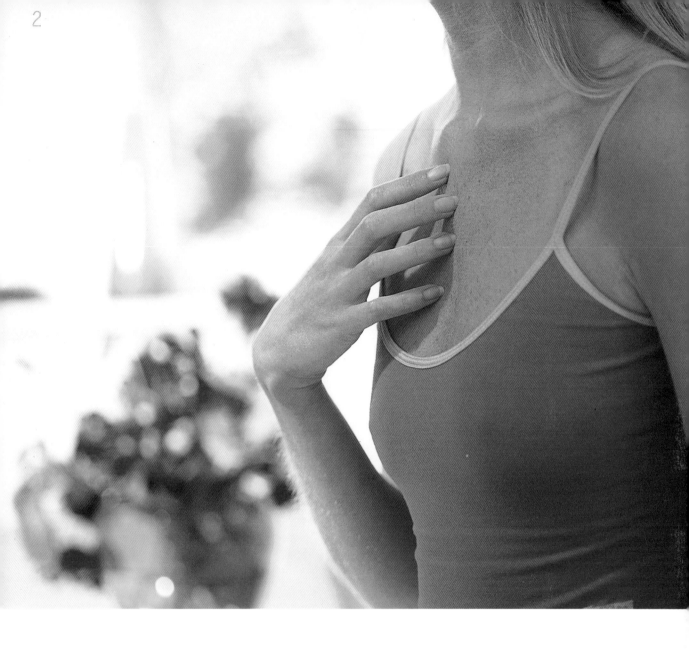

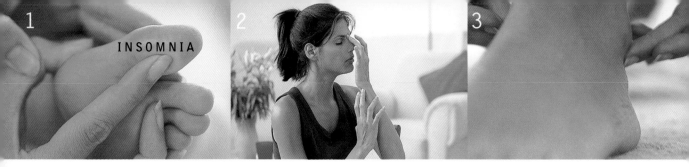

INSOMNIA

As so often happens, energy therapies work best in conjunction with life style changes. Try to empty your mind of worries before you go to bed. Listen to a relaxation tape or soothing music. Establish a calming routine every night, such as a warm aromatherapy bath, a cup of camomile tea, putting out clothes for the next day, or a relaxation exercise. If you can't sleep, get up and read in another room until you feel drowsy. However do make sure that your reading matter is not disturbing.

Reflexology

First work on the brain and central nervous system, then the entire spine, to relieve the underlying tension that frequently disturbs sleep. Next, work on the pineal gland (1), which helps to balance the biorhythms, particularly if the problem is caused by jet lag. Work on the pituitary gland to regulate hormones and the adrenal glands, solar plexus and diaphragm to reduce stress.

Acupressure

Treatment depends on the cause of sleeplessness. If it is what traditional Chinese medicine would see as an overactive organ or chi stagnation, you may need to work on opening the channel with a meridian massage. If you have become hyperactive this could be the gall bladder, or the liver if you have been eating too much fatty food. If you are overexcited, work on the heart meridian and use H7 (2). If your heart is burdened with worries, talking things through with a friend may help as well.

For general help with sleep, massage the 'third eye' point (2). Or rub the insides and outsides of your heels, to work on Ki 6, also known as 'close eyes', and Bl 62, 'calm sleep' (3). Surprisingly, Ki 6 (on the opposite side of the heel from Bl 62) can also have the opposite effect and help you keep your eyes open when you are tired.

COUGHS, COLDS, CHEST PROBLEMS

One of the easiest ways to avoid infections is, believe it or not, to wash your hands more often, including every time you come in from outside. It really does reduce the number of germs that reach your face and hence your lungs. A gram or so of Vitamin C a day can stop a cold, or at least make it milder, if you take it as soon as you get the first inkling of symptoms – although too large a dose can sometimes cause diarrhoea.

It is always a good idea to drink plenty of water after you have had a reflexology session. Even more so if you have a cold or chest infection, because you are losing a lot of fluid: some of the miserable symptoms are signs of dehydration. And extra water stimulates the kidneys to carry away any toxins.

Reflexology

Work deliberately and thoroughly over the whole lung area, noticing any crunchiness. To ease a sore throat, work the front and sides of the big toe below the nail – the throat area with your finger (1). Don't forget the thymus reflex, to help dry up the snuffles. To work the lymph nodes in the throat and neck, massage with circular movements between and beneath the toes. Rubbing gently down the sides of the toes (2) will encourage the sinuses to drain. Then gently draw your index finger from the base of each toe down into the chest area. If you are working on the hand 'milk' the area below the fingers in order to drain the lymph nodes (3).

Chest problems may arise if the body isn't getting rid of toxins through the normal routes, the kidney and bowels, so work on the abdomen and urinary systems too. On the left foot, do some extra work on the spleen to stimulate the immune system. Work on the ileocaecal valve reflex to normalise mucus secretion.

Acupressure

For coughs and colds, work on point Ki 27 (4). Massage with oil on the upper back beside the spine along Bl 11 to 13. For bronchitis and emphysema, give a stimulating massage to Lung 1 on the upper chest.

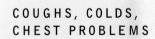

**COUGHS, COLDS,
CHEST PROBLEMS**

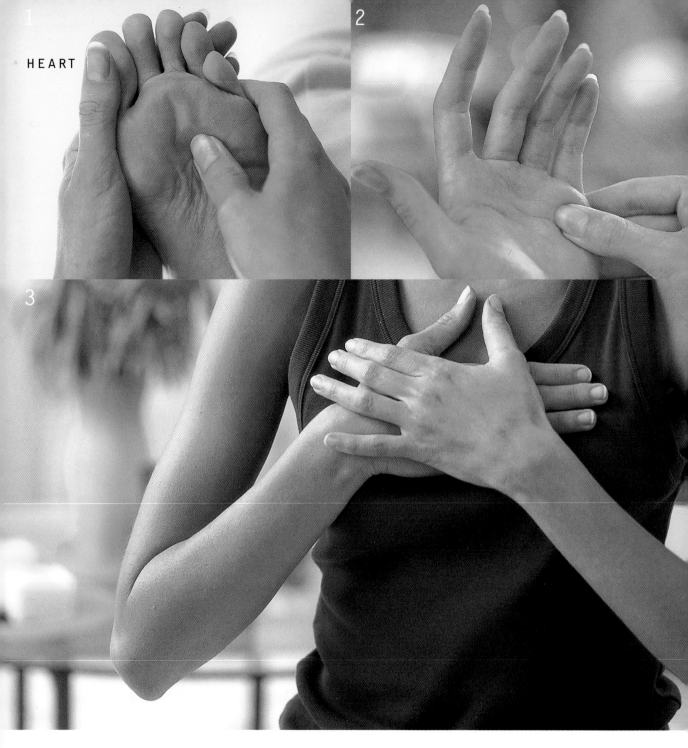

HEART

Giving up smoking is the best thing you can do for your heart, so try to find something you like better and spend the money you save on that instead. Food supplements have been shown to have unexpectedly strong effects on heart conditions: the main ones are 1–2g of vitamin C, 100–400IU (or 100–400mg) natural vitamin E (d-alpha-tocopherol, not dl-alpha-tocopherol) and a daily vitamin B complex supplement; choose one that contains about 400mcg of folic acid. Stress is almost as bad for the heart as smoking, so make stress-reduction a priority. Meditation and breathing exercises can also help.

Reflexology

To strengthen the heart, it is preferable to carry out an entire reflexology session, since you need to try to divert energy away from the surface to support the heart. In a shorter routine, work on the respiratory system as well as the cardiac (1, 2), to improve the supply of oxygen.

Warning: if there is any danger of thrombosis, don't do reflexology. It is known to stimulate the circulation, and you don't want to risk moving a blood clot. Check with your GP, since in some cases it may be safe to work very lightly and gently – but do make sure your GP knows the effects of reflexology.

Acupressure

To calm the heart, slowly and gently rub the centre of your chest around the heart point CV 17 (3) with your palm while breathing out and letting your mind and shoulders relax. Heart problems can also be eased by working on both the heart and the small intestine meridians.

VARICOSE VEINS

Standing for a long time causes the blood to pool in the legs, so if you have to stay on your feet, move around as much as possible. If you are sitting a lot, don't cross your legs. Keep circling your ankles and wriggling your toes to help circulation.

Reflexology

Work on the eliminatory system, since this condition is often exacerbated by constipation. Add the heart (since this is a circulatory problem), the adrenal glands, the diaphragm and solar plexus and the arm and shoulder for a cross-reflex action. And of course work the lower legs – the outer edge of the foot from the knee point below the bump towards the heel (1).

Acupressure

Work on Sp 9 on the other leg. If the varicose veins are in both legs, use the lightest pressure on Sp 9. Work on the points that aid the heart, in order to strengthen the circulatory system.

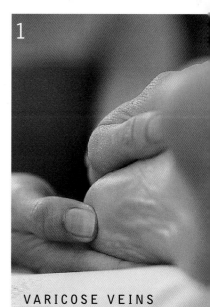

VARICOSE VEINS

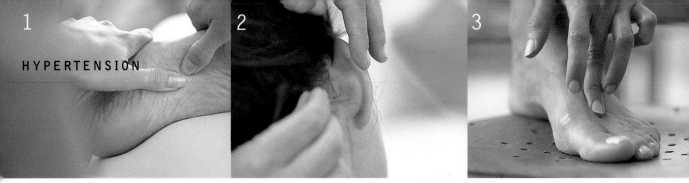

HYPERTENSION

HYPERTENSION (HIGH BLOOD PRESSURE)

Meditation has had such good effects on blood pressure that some doctors prescribe a course of it. Cutting down on salt makes a big difference too – most salt is hidden in processed foods, so eating more fresh fruit and vegetables will reduce your salt intake naturally.

Reflexology

Work on the diaphragm, cervical vertebrae, adrenals (1), stomach and gall bladder. A full treatment will be particularly helpful.

Acupressure

Pinch all around the edge of the earlobe and behind the ear where it meets the head, pressing into the back of the ear (2). Find Liv 3 – between the big and second toes, two finger-widths down the top of the foot from the bottom of the toe – and press it to reduce hypertension (3). Don't press too hard, or the blood pressure could drop too far.

PROBLEMS OF MIDLIFE AND BEYOND

Staying physically active, eating well and keeping up outside interests are the key to ageing in a healthy condition. While drugs can be life-saving for serious problems that resist other treatments, using reflexology and acupressure for minor ailments keeps you off the health-sapping roundabout of unnecessary drugs and their side effects and possible adverse reactions. Remember to treat ageing skin and joints gently.

Reflexology

Work on the head and neck system to protect your sight and hearing as well as mental alacrity. If you start noting signs of problems such as constipation or incontinence, add the entire eliminatory and urinary systems too. If you don't have time for full foot treatments, make a decision to spend a little while working on one system at a time, covering the whole body every few weeks.

   If you start getting ringing in the ears – tinnitus – pinch the Eustachian tube point, which is located in the webbing between the third and fourth fingers (1) or toes, if you are working on the feet.

To improve your balance, and if you suffer from vertigo, work the balance point at the bottom of the fourth finger (2) or toe, on the side next to the little finger or toe, using a hook and back-up move.

Acupressure

Walking fairly long distances keeps bones strong and stimulates Ki 1 for energy. Several acupressure points can be pressed or massaged to help improve memory: GV 26, GB 20, the heart point CV 17 and the 'third eye'.

Massaging the great yang point in the temples, the dip just beside the outer edge of the eyes, sharpens concentration as well as being a natural way of easing headaches. Do the meridian massages every day to keep all your systems strong and balanced.

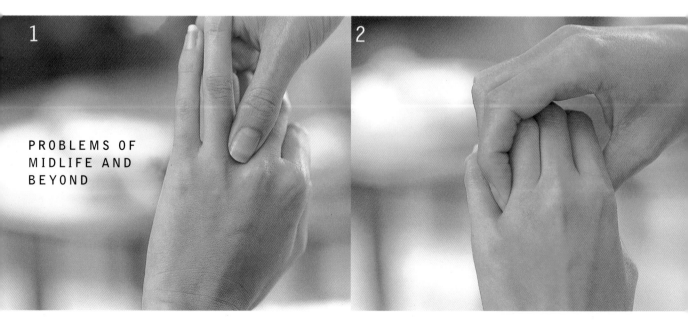

1

2

PROBLEMS OF
MIDLIFE AND
BEYOND

the inner self

Reflexology and acupressure are as beneficial for the mind as the body. We tend to overlook the mind in our busy lives, even though stress is a major health hazard. So it is well worth taking a little time for a relaxing or revitalising treatment to keep the energies flowing smoothly.

INCREASING ENERGY

You don't have to be tired out before you start working on increasing your energy levels. After all, you wouldn't wait until you were fainting before you would eat, or until you were seriously ill before you would start caring for your health. Energy therapies such as reflexology and acupressure are about putting your whole self into balance, so why not use them to enhance good health?

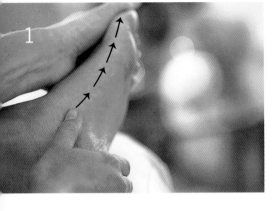

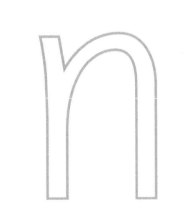

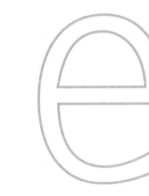

Reflexology

Spend extra time on the relaxing and the preparatory techniques. Continue by working on the brain and the central nervous system, including the spine (1), the endocrine system, kidneys and pancreas, as well as the diaphragm and the solar plexus.

Acupressure

To enhance your immune system and increase vitality, work on Sp 21 – but be gentle, since the area can be sensitive. Do this quite often, three or four times a day for best effect. In addition, work on the points TE 5 and LI 11, the 'great energiser' (2).

When you are tired, rub your palms together to activate Pc 8 and then press them on Ki 1, which is located on the sole of the foot.

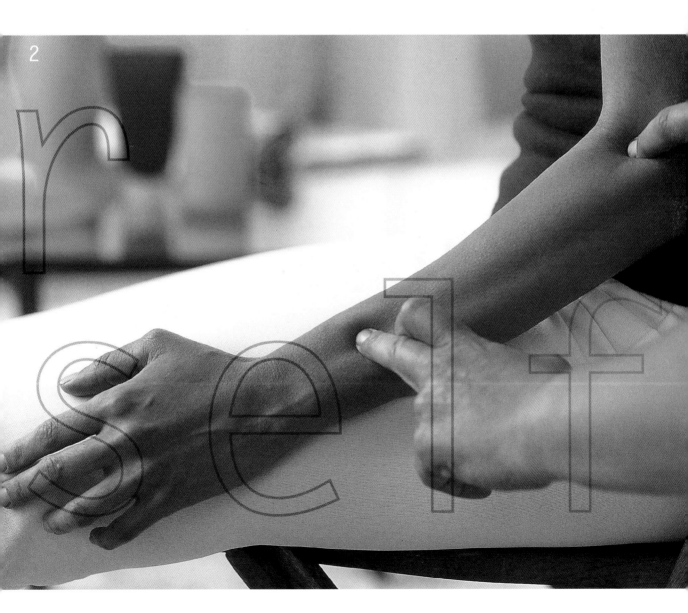

DEPRESSION

It is important not to let depression become a habit. If you can't shake off your low mood, try to identify and solve problems that are keeping you down. Since this may take time, make sure you are seeing friends, doing things you enjoy and – most important – taking some energetic exercise at least three times a week. Counselling may help, and the herbal remedy St John's wort has proved to be effective in easing mild to moderate depression. If necessary, your doctor may prescribe a short course of antidepressants (unlike tranquillisers, they are not addictive), which can break the pattern long enough to help you get back on your feet. Don't hesitate to see your GP if you feel you are losing hope.

Reflexology

Start with the brain and central nervous system, then work on the kidneys (which are believed to be the site of

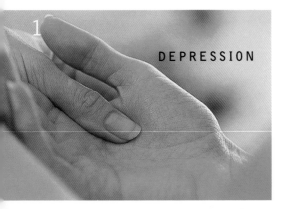

1

DEPRESSION

suppressed tears), the adrenals (1) to lift exhaustion, the neck to relieve tension and the solar plexus to increase energy. Work on the pylorus and ileocaecal valve to stimulate the digestive system, which often becomes sluggish when you are depressed.

Acupressure

Body tension and poor posture can contribute to depression. Work on the spleen meridian to 'earth' yourself. Chinese philosophy links depression with thinking too much, so give yourself a break. Rub up and down the fleshy sides of the lower legs from the knee to the ankle, inside and outside, to stimulate Sp 4–10 and St 40 (2).

Lung 7 and Lung 10 are good points for releasing stagnation, allowing blocked energy to move and freeing repressed emotions. Lung points are affected by grief.

ANXIETY AND STRESS

The breathing technique described at the beginning of Soothing Pain (page 87) is also useful for relieving anxiety. If you frequently suffer from this, find some stress-reducing activity that works for you. Among the most effective are walking, meditation, vigorous exercise, relaxation tapes, talking matters through with friends and taking practical action to remove the sources of stress.

Reflexology

After working the chest and abdomen, do some extra work on the solar plexus and diaphragm to encourage relaxation, and on the adrenals to relieve stress. A valuable stress-relieving technique is to grip your fingers until you feel a pulse. Hold the thumb firmly in your other hand to relieve worry (1), the index finger for fear, the middle finger for anger, the ring finger for sadness and the little finger if you have been trying too hard.

Acupressure

Work Liv 3, LI 4 and H 7. Be conscious of your posture when you are stressed: muscle tension can hunch you up, leading to pain and internal problems. Stretch your spine. Do some breathing exercises while touching the 'sea of energy' CV 6 (2), two finger-widths below the navel, to bring energy down, or while gently massaging the heart point CV 17 (2). When worried, rub the stomach both clockwise and anticlockwise or have the inside border of the shoulder blade massaged (3).

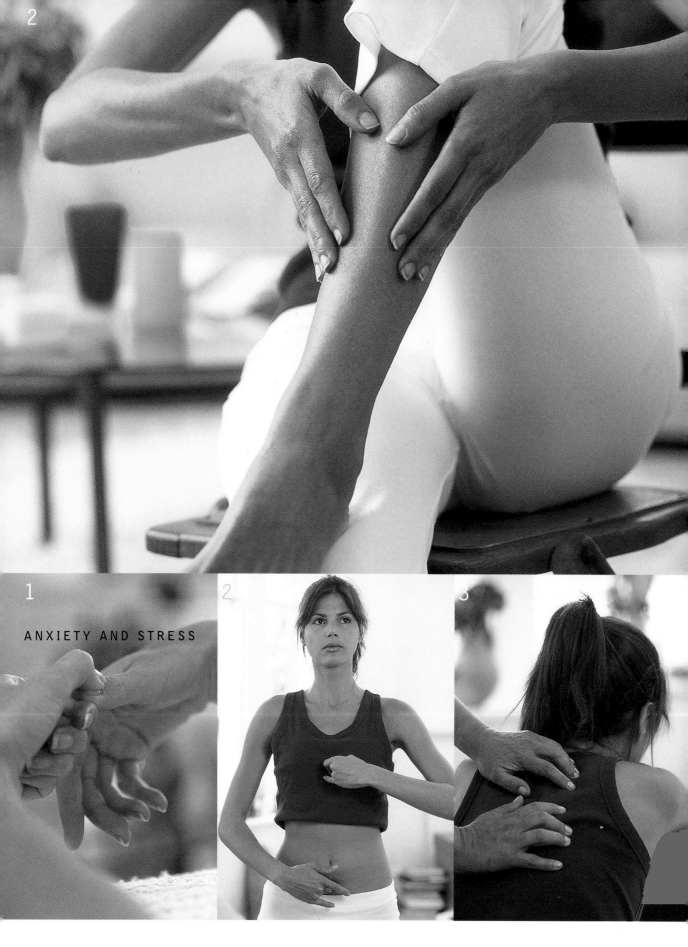

2

ANXIETY AND STRESS

1

2

3

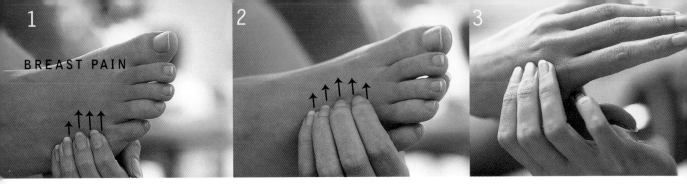

women's conditions

The conditions that women are prone to suffer from do not often respond to orthodox medical treatment. However, the symptoms frequently associated with menstruation, childbirth and the menopause can often be alleviated by using reflexology and acupressure.

BREAST PAIN AND LUMPS

About 20 per cent of all women find that their breasts become painful and lumpy before a period. (If you ever notice a lump that does not go away, see your doctor as soon as possible.) Cutting down on caffeine often relieves the discomfort. Evening primrose oil has been proved to help many women – the usual recommended dosage is six to eight 500mg capsules a day. However, you do have to persevere; it may take up to three months for the effects to show. Up to 100mg a day of Vitamin B6 has also proved beneficial (the current EU Recommended Daily Allowance for supplements is 2mg a day).

Warning: do not take evening primrose oil if you suffer from epilepsy.

Reflexology

Work the entire lymphatic system, paying special attention to the reflexes for the lymph glands that are in the armpits (1), especially the left one, which does most of the work. Gently rub up and down the breast area on the top of the foot (2), covering a couple of centimetres from the base of the toes.

Alternatively, massage the breast area on the hand, which is located between the thumb and forefinger (3).

Acupressure

For help with problems such as mastitis, swollen breasts or fluid retention, massage the TE meridian downwards (open), tapping along its route from the head to the ring finger, since this meridian balances the fluid levels between the kidney and the heart (or, in the terminology of orthodox medicine, it stimulates the lymph system).

PREMENSTRUAL SYNDROME (PMS)

Food causes more hormonal problems than it was once thought. To ease mood swings and tension, try eating more foods rich in vitamin B6, such as fish, liver, bacon, yeast extract – Marmite is a good source – tomato purée and bananas, and magnesium, found in muesli, oatmeal, dried fruit and dried skimmed milk. Wholemeal bread, soya flour, mung beans and nuts contain plenty of both. Eat little and often before a period, and cut down on fatty foods to keep hormone levels as stable as possible.

Reflexology

Start with the entire lymphatic (1) and reproductive systems, including the fallopian tubes (2), following these with the endocrine system to ensure normal hormonal activity. In particular, hook onto the pituitary gland (3) in the centre of the thumb or big toe pad. Next work the eliminatory system, paying special attention to the kidneys in order to combat fluid retention, and the colon if you have a tendency to constipation. If PMS causes headaches, add the head and brain. Working on the solar plexus will aid relaxation.

Self-help is invaluable when you have PMS; working on your hands is soothing and accessible at any time of day. Work the uterus below the thumb just above the bump of bone, the ovaries below the little fingers and the fallopian tubes across the back of the wrist.

Acupressure

Massage the spleen meridian and St 29.

PMS

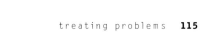

1

HEAVY OR PAINFUL
PERIODS

2

3

1

CYSTITIS AND THRUSH

HEAVY OR PAINFUL PERIODS

If you have heavy periods make sure you are getting enough iron in your diet to replace what you are losing. But do not take supplements unless your GP prescribes them. Drink orange juice with meals to help you absorb the iron from food, and wait several hours before drinking milk, as calcium and iron compete with each other. Other foods rich in iron include offal such as liver and kidneys, dried apricots, cocoa, sardines and fortified breakfast cereals.

Reflexology

Heavy and painful periods are best treated with an entire reflexology session, since the reproductive system is low on the body's priority list for energy and will benefit from toning up the whole system. Alternatively – or having completed the overall treatment – work on the whole endocrine and reproductive systems, then pay extra attention to the uterus (1), ovaries, pituitary and spine, including the lower back area (2). Also work on the kidneys and ureter to remove any stress from other organs in that area.

Acupressure

Work on points on the lower back, such as Bl 23 to 29 (3): put your hands on your waist, pressing your thumbs into the long muscles beside your spine, starting at waist level and working your way down to your hips. For extra effect, rotate your hips as you are pressing. Also, put the backs of your hands on your lower back to connect the bladder meridian with LI 4, calming and opening the circulation in that area. Heat on the small of the back can prevent pain: use a hot water bottle if this feels right. For heavy periods, rub the breasts to bring energy up and stimulate the hormone prolactin. Lying on juggling balls to massage your back (see page 77) is bliss for lower back ache. Rubbing Sp 12 and Sp 13, in the groin crease at the front top of the thigh, can ease menstrual pain. And CV 6, below the navel, can regulate periods and ease cramps.

CYSTITIS AND THRUSH

The thick discharge of thrush and painful urination caused by cystitis are common nuisances that thrive on anything that irritates the vulva and vagina. If you are prone to these problems, wash in lukewarm water, don't use harsh soaps or bubble baths and never use vaginal deodorants or douches, which can harm the healthiest system. Avoid the warm, moist conditions created by hot baths, nylon underwear, tights and tight trousers.

If you do get cystitis, drink large quantities of unsweetened cranberry juice or, if you can get hold of them, a tea made from cherry stalks; otherwise drink plenty of water just to dilute the burning urine. See your GP if cystitis lasts more than three days, since it can lead to a serious kidney infection.

Reflexology

Work the entire urinary system, then concentrate on the kidneys, bladder, ureter (1), vagina and urethra. Also work on the adrenals, abdomen and lower back and on the lower parts of the lymphatic system to combat infection.

Acupressure

Work on St 29. A general point for anything to do with women's problems is Sp 6.

Warning: do not use Sp 6 during pregnancy.

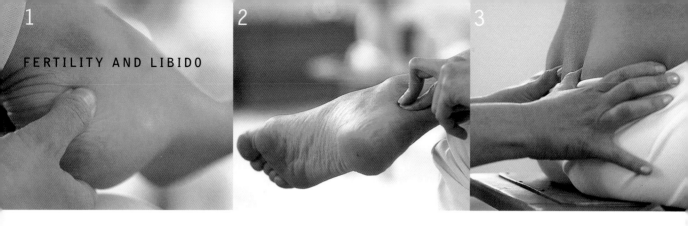

FERTILITY AND LIBIDO

FERTILITY AND LIBIDO

Our sexual appetites wax and wane quite naturally, and we all go through periods when we are more interested in other things. Stress, exhaustion, depression and conflict are also common causes for loss of libido.

Reflexology

Work on the entire reproductive and endocrine systems, then concentrate on the reflexes for the sexual organs: the ovaries (1), uterus and fallopian tubes.

Acupressure

Work on Ki 3 (2). Stimulate the back and the adrenal area Bl 23, Bl 27 to 29 and 31 to 33 (3). Massage CV 6, just below the navel, to increase fertility. Massage your back by lying on a couple of juggling balls, wedged just beside your spine.

PREGNANCY

These simple remedies are ideal for partners to learn, to help women through pregnancy and childbirth.

Warning : don't use reflexology in the first 16 weeks of pregnancy in case the changed flow of energy triggers a miscarriage, especially in a first pregnancy or if the woman has miscarried before.

Reflexology

If miscarriage is a low risk, you can work lightly on yourself during the early stages. Morning sickness can be treated as other kinds of sickness: start by working the whole digestive system, concentrating on the oesophagus to ease nausea (1), using hand reflexology if you are doing this for yourself so that you don't have to cramp your stomach while working your foot. Return to the solar plexus and pituitary gland points, rotating your thumb on them. Thumb-walk across the diaphragm and the middle and upper spine, and work some strips over the stomach area. Because morning sickness is caused by the hormonal changes of pregnancy, include the endocrine system to help balance hormones.

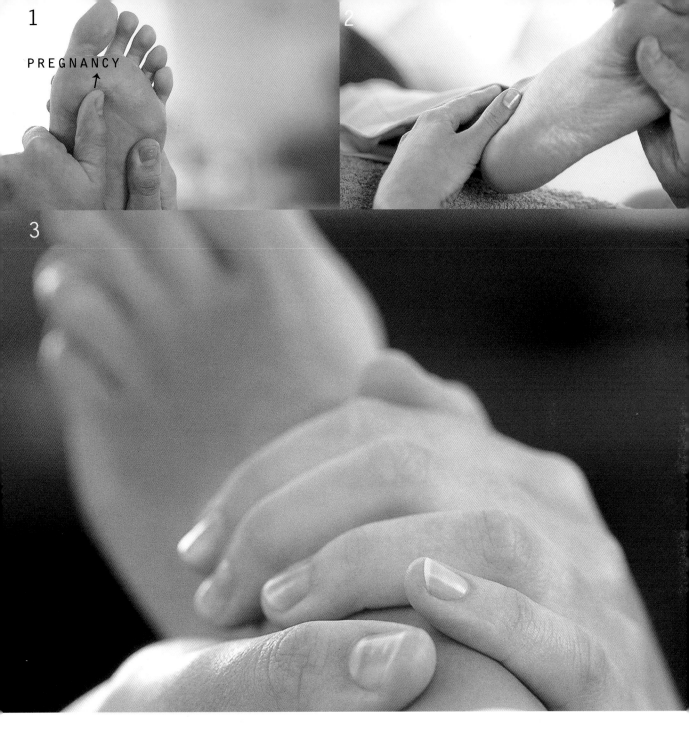

PREGNANCY

Later in the pregnancy reflexology is a boon for easing aching legs and back (2): work on the reproductive and musculo-skeletal systems. A gentle foot massage is very soothing and suited to the later stages of pregnancy (3).

Acupressure

Pc 6 is a reliable remedy for morning sickness. Rubbing up and down the conception channel below the navel helps maintain a pregnancy if there was difficulty conceiving.

Warning : don't overwork the uterus and pituitary gland until the last days of pregnancy. Don't use Sp 6 in pregnancy.

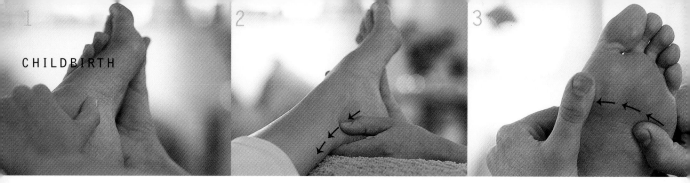

CHILDBIRTH

Try to have your birth plan organised well in advance in case the baby arrives earlier than expected. Also, try to ensure the attending staff are sympathetic to your wishes – for example if you don't want routine interventions.

Reflexology

Studies have shown that women who received reflexology during pregnancy have a shorter and more comfortable labour. During labour, treat the middle and lower back reflexes (1), and concentrate on giving a relaxing foot massage with plenty of long, smooth effleurage strokes.

Reflexology is particularly of benefit when preparing to give birth. During the last two weeks of pregnancy, work on the entire reproductive system and pay special attention to the breasts and adrenals. If the due date passes, work on the uterus, the 'chronic helper' (2) at the back of the Achilles tendon, and the pituitary to encourage the birth process to start.

After the birth, work on the endocrine and reproductive systems along with the adrenals. Follow up with a series of treatments to normalise hormone levels and help get the muscles back into shape. Working on the endocrine system will enhance breastfeeding. Reflexology can also help the body recover after a caesarean.

Try to give full treatments as much as possible. In addition to the healing benefits of reflexology, any kind of caring attention to a new mother can help prevent postnatal depression and give her a chance to bond peacefully with the baby.

Postnatal depression may respond well to working on the endocrine and reproductive systems, the adrenals and, to aid relaxation, the diaphragm (3) and solar plexus.

Acupressure

To prevent premature birth, work on Ki 3 while tightening the pelvic floor. During birth, massage Bl 27 at the side of the sacrum and Sp 6 and Sp 9 (4) on the inside of the knees between pushes. Sp 6 could help speed labour. Electronic acupressure (TENS) has proved to ease the pain of childbirth. For a healthy milk supply, massage St 29, the whole of TE meridian and the heart point, CV 17.

MENOPAUSE

This can be a time of liberating, exhilarating change. Some women even find that hot flushes – or 'power surges' – clear their heads. Eating soy products, from health-food companies that don't use genetically modified soy, may help keep the hormones in balance and reduce any unwelcome symptoms.

Reflexology

This is another time when a full treatment works wonders, both for the benefits to all the body's systems and for the relaxing effects of a complete foot massage, taking time out for yourself. Work on the reproductive and endocrine systems, including the thyroid (1), to help yourself or a friend through the transition. Next, pay attention to the uterus (2), 'chronic helper', ovaries, liver and the eliminatory parts of the digestive and urinary systems to prevent constipation.

Acupressure

For hot flushes, work on Sp 6, Liv 3 and Pc 6. If these don't help, acupuncture may. Remember to exercise; dancing is excellent and stamping your feet helps to build bones, reducing the risk of osteoporosis. If you have a ribbed wooden foot roller, use this to massage your feet.

Work on Sp 6, four finger-widths up the inner leg from the ankle bone, starting from the fleshy area behind the ankle bone. Work on Ki 1 (3) while rotating the ankle. Walking stimulates Ki 1 as well as being an excellent form of exercise, all of which makes a daily walk particularly valuable at this time of life. Rotating the ankle whilst holding Ki 1 in the palm of the hand can invigorate the body.

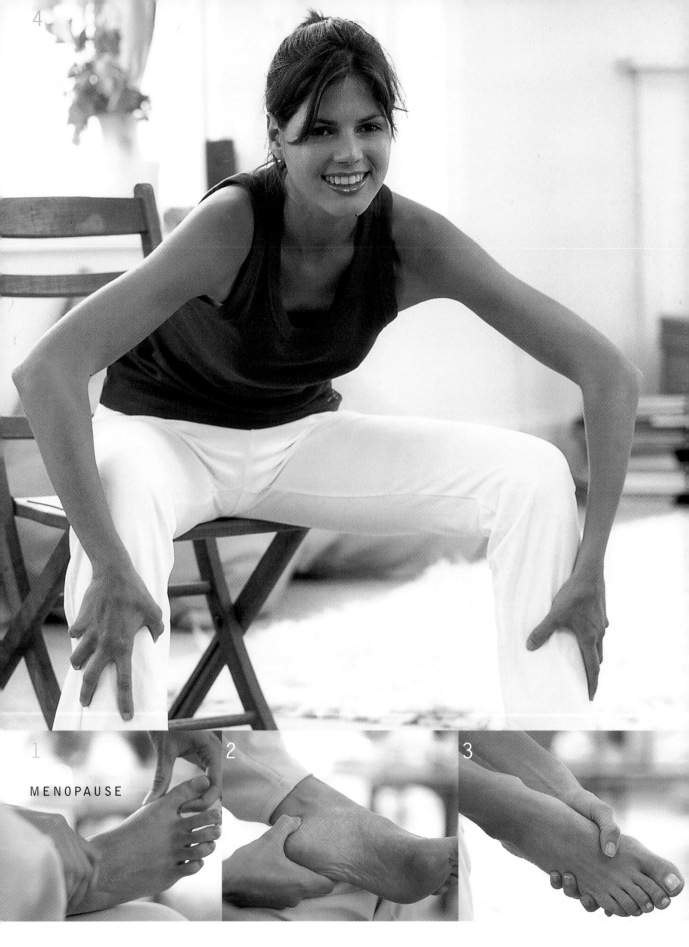

4

1

MENOPAUSE

2

3

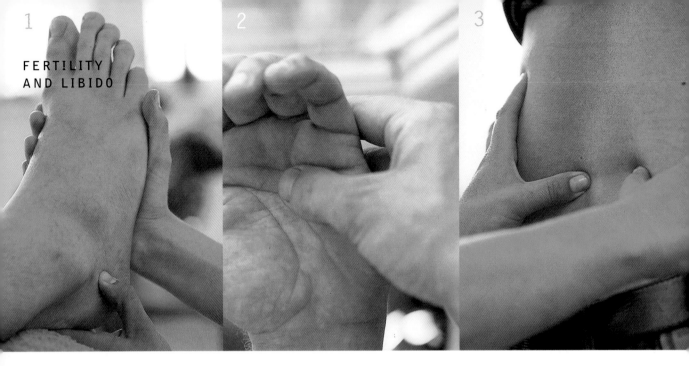

men's conditions

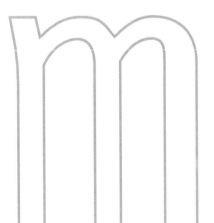

Fertility in men and women has declined alarmingly over the past few decades. Stress, overwork, smoking and chemical pollution may be responsible, as well as sabotaging our general health.

FERTILITY AND LIBIDO

Tension and anxiety are behind many problems in this area, so find enough time for relaxation and having fun. Exercise and a healthy diet with plenty of fresh vegetables and fruit help your body to function at full capacity. They will also reduce any excess weight. Sperm thrives in a cool environment, so avoid tight pants and very hot baths.

Reflexology

As for women, work on the entire reproductive and endocrine systems, then concentrate on the reflexes for the sexual organs: testes (1), prostate and vas deferens. Include the diaphragm (2) and solar plexus to reduce counter-productive tension.

Acupressure

Work Ki 3. Stimulate the back and adrenal area Bl 23 (3), Bl 27 to 29 and 31 to 33. Use juggling balls to massage the small of your back (see page 77), working on points that increase sexual energy, including Bl 23.

Work on Liv 8, which is located inside the knees. Sp 6 can improve libido. Pressing and holding the 'sea of energy' spot, CV 6, situated below the navel, can help to counteract both impotence and low fertility.

PROTECTING THE PROSTATE

Prostate disorders are common as men get older, although most are more of a nuisance than a serious health risk. Cutting down on fatty foods and drinking plenty of water during the day can help; these also reduce the likelihood of constipation, which aggravates prostate problems.

Reflexology

Work on the endocrine, urinary and reproductive systems (1), then work the lower spine and the 'chronic helper' on the Achilles' heel.

Acupressure

Massaging beside the spine from the waist down relieves many male problems, especially in older age.

MALE MENOPAUSE

Problems at this time of life often have a psychological basis, especially if men have been made redundant (or just feel that way). But there's some evidence that changing hormone levels also play a part, as with women.

Reflexology

Work on the endocrine and reproductive systems, including the vas deferens (1), to balance hormone levels, along with the lower back. Add the diaphragm and solar plexus to reduce stress, the eliminatory organs and urinary system including the bladder (2), the liver and the 'chronic helper'.

Acupressure

Sp 6 is a valuable energy point when men are feeling low in libido or vitality. Work on Liv 8, rubbing the inner side of the knee. To alleviate worries about testosterone diminishing, work on St 36 – a good point for hormone balancing and for energy. To slow the rate of hair loss, stimulate the scalp with gentle head massage, without pulling the roots, and work on the kidney meridian.

Knee injuries are common: use the acupressure treatment for knee pain to release excess energy trapped in this area. Rubbing the inside of the knee, a yin area including Liv 8, encourages the flow of calming yin energy, balancing excessive yang energy in men who are aggressive and stressed.

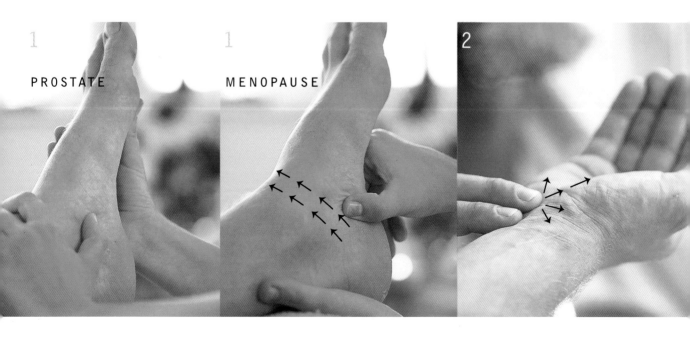

1   PROSTATE   1   MENOPAUSE   2

glossary

ALEXANDER TECHNIQUE – a process of re-education, which aims to teach us to rediscover our natural posture and use our bodies more efficiently. It can help relieve stress-related conditions, breathing disorders and neck and joint pain.

CHAKRAS – energy centres, taken from a sanskrit word meaning 'wheel'. There are seven chakras in the body: in the sacral region, abdomen, solar plexus, heart, throat, brow and crown of the head, roughly corresponding to the part of the body in which they are situated.

CHI – according to Eastern medical theory, chi energy is carried to every part of the body by the meridian channels.

FELDENKRAIS – a process for improving body awareness with gentle, non-strenuous movements. It can help to relieve stress as well as improving general posture and soothing chronic pain.

HOMEOSTASIS – the body's self-healing mechanism which strives to rectify health problems and balance the body. If the self-healing mechanism is not working correctly it can lead to dysfunction and possible disease.

MERIDIANS – chi circulates around the body in meridian vessels. There are 14 main meridians, twelve of which are connected to one of the internal organs and have a greater effect on that organ. The remaining two are the governor vessel, which runs up the spine and over the head, and the conception vessel which runs up the centre front of the body.

MOXIBUSTION – coming from the Japanese word 'mocusa', meaning burning herb, moxibustion works by stimulating pressure points with heat.

TRIPLE ENERGISER – traditional Chinese term used to describe the three body cavities which comprise the chest, abdomen and lower abdomen.

PLACEBO – medication or treatment prescribed for psychological reasons but having no physiological effect. A placebo may be used as a control in scientific trials.

YANG – the male principle of Chinese philosophy, representing positivity, activity, heat, light, vigour, day and Summer.

YIN – the female principle of Chinese philosophy, representing negativity, passivity, cold, dark, stillness, night, Winter.

useful addresses

Contact one of these addresses to find a qualified practitioner in your area, or for information about training courses. Acupuncture organisations also cover acupressurists.

The Institute for Complementary Medicine, PO Box 194, London SE16 1QZ, UK, tel 0171-237 5165 (SAE and two loose stamps). Keeps the British Register of Complementary Practitioners, a database of practitioners of various complementary therapies who have passed the ICM's own exams, marked by independent assessors.

The British Complementary Medicine Association, 39 Prestbury Road, Pittville, Cheltenham, Glos GL52 2PT, UK, tel 01242-226770. An umbrella group for numerous therapies including reflexology and acupressure.

International Federation of Reflexology, 76–78 Edridge Rd, Croydon, Surrey CR0 1EF, 0181-667 9458. Keeps a computer database of qualified reflexologists from various schools.

Association of Reflexologists, 27 Old Gloucester Street, London WC1N 3XX, tel 0870-567 3320. Trains and keeps a register of reflexologists who have met its requirements.

Holistic Association of Reflexologists (and British School of Reflexology), 92 Sheering Road, Old Harlow, Essex CN17 0JW, 01279-429060. Trains and keeps a register of reflexologists who have met its requirements.

British Medical Acupuncture Society, Newton House, Newton Lane, Whitley, Warrington, Cheshire, 01925-730727. Doctors of medicine who have also trained in acupuncture.

The Acupuncture Association of Chartered Physiotherapists, Abbey View Complementary Clinic, The Medical Centre, Shaftesbury, Dorset SP7 8DH, tel 01747-850784. Usefully combining in-depth knowledge of the body from the Western as well as the Chinese viewpoint, practitioners are fully qualified in physiotherapy as well as acupuncture.

The British Acupuncture Council, Park House, 206 Latimer Road, London W10 6RE, tel 0181-964 0222. <www. acupuncture.org.uk> An umbrella group covering a large number of practitioners.

index

acknowledgements

Publishing Director: **Laura Bamford**
Executive Editor: **Jane McIntosh**
Project Editor: **Catharine Davey**
Editor: **Casey Horton**
Consultant Therapists: **B.K. Heather** (Reflexology)
                       Sara Mokone (Acupressure)
Therapists appearing
in photography: **Nikki Corrigan** (Reflexology)
                Sara Mokone (Acupressure)
Models: **Susan Alston**
        Maria Rodreguez
Stylist: **Leeann Mackenzie**
Picture Researcher: **Zoë Holtermann**
Production Controller: **Karina Han**
Indexer: **Hilary Flenley**

Creative Director: **Keith Martin**
Design Manager: **Bryan Dunn**
Designer: **Vivek Bhatia**
Photographer: **Ian Wallace**
Illustrators: **Peter Gerrish**
              Annabel Milne (pages **6–7**)

First published in Great Britain in 1999 by Hamlyn,
a division of Octopus Publishing Group Limited, 2–4
Heron Quays, London, E14 4JP
Reprinted 1999, 2001

ISBN 0 600 59682 6

A CIP catalogue record of this book is available
from the British Library.

Picture credits in source order:
The Publishers would like to thank the following individuals and
organizations for their kind permission to reproduce photographs in
this book. While every effort has been made to acknowledge
copyright holders we would like to apologize should there have been
any omissions.

Bridgeman Art Library, London, New York/Freud Museum, London,
UK 22, /National Museum of India, New Delhi, India 18
Corbis UK Ltd/Dean Conger 20, /Owen Franken 21
E.T. Archive 13, 19
London Library/From the 'Golden Mirror' 11 Bottom, /From: 'Ling
Shu Su Wen Chieh' 10, /From: 'Ling Shu Su Wen Chieh' Yee 11 Top
Octopus Publishing Group Ltd/Ian Wallace Front Cover, Back Cover,
Front flap, Back flap, Front Endpaper, Back Endpaper, 1, 2 left, 2
right, 3 left, 3 right, 4 Top Left, 4 Top Right, 4 Bottom, 8–9, 9 Top
Right, 9 Bottom Right, 16–17, 17 Top Right, 17 Bottom Right,
24–25, 25 Top Right, 25 Bottom Right, 26, 27, 28, 29, 30, 31,
32–33, 33, 33 Top Right, 34, 35, 36 Bottom Left, 36 Bottom Right,
37 Bottom Left, 37 Bottom Right, 38 Top, 39 Top, 39 Bottom, 40,
41, 42, 43, 44, 45, 47 Top, 47 Bottom, 48, 49, 50, 51, 52, 53, 54,
55, 56, 57, 58, 59, 60, 61, 62–63, 63, 63 Top, 64, 65 left, 65 right,
66, 67, 69, 70 Top, 70 Bottom Left, 70 Bottom Right, 72, 73 Top,
73 Bottom Left, 73 Bottom Right, 74 Top, 74 Bottom, 75 left, 75
right, 76 left, 76 right, 77, 78–79, 79, 79 Top, 80, 81, 82, 83, 84
Top Left, 84 Top Right, 84 Bottom, 85, 86, 87, 88, 89 left, 89 right,
90, 91, 92, 93, 94, 95, 96, 97, 98, 99, 100, 101, 102, 103, 104,
105, 106, 107, 108, 109, 110, 111, 112, 113 Top, 113 Bottom,
114, 115, 116 Top, 116 Bottom, 118, 119, 120, 121 Top, 121
Bottom, 122, 123 Bottom Left, 123 Bottom Centre, 123 Bottom
Right
Photographed by Paolo Scremin/ © Oxford Expedition To Egypt 23
Wellcome Institute Library, London 15
Werner Forman Archive/Haiphong Museum, Vietnam 12